THE SCIENTIFIC APPROACH TO INTERMITTENT FASTING

The Scientific Approach to Intermittent Fasting

Find out how a simple lifestyle change can completely transform your health and life!

Dr. Michael VanDerschelden

The Scientific Approach to
Intermittent Fasting

Ordering Information:
Quantity sales. Special discounts are available on quantity purchases by
corporations, associations, and others. For details, contact the author at
drmichaelvan@gmail.com

Printed in the United States of America
Edited by: Tiffany Avans

Associated Websites:
drmichaelvan.com
drmichaelvan.com/5

Videos/Lectures:
youtube.com/drmichaelvandc

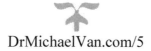

CONTENTS

INTRODUCTION

"The people who say they don't have time to take care of themselves will soon discover they're spending all their time being sick."   - Patricia Alexander

I see it happen too many times. January 1st is approaching, and you begin to think of what your healthy New Years resolutions are going to be this year; 99% of the time they will revolve around your physical aesthetics. They are mostly centered around losing fat, gaining muscle, and losing weight. One might say, "I'm going to diet and lose 20 lbs." "I'm going to workout and get ripped." "I'm going to lose 5% of my mid-section belly fat." You realize that you ate an abundance of junk food with too little exercise all year long, especially during the holiday seasons. You begin to sense your health is getting out of control, and become poised to make a change.

Do these resolutions of healthy living and healthy eating work? I think we all know that answer to that question. If they did, you wouldn't have to make health your New Years resolution each and every year. If you have recently made a commitment to lose weight and get healthy, was that the first time you did so? Or are you like the rest of the people out there and made that same commitment to yourself a countless number of times, only to find that you keep ending up at square one where you initially started.

Everyone wants to lose weight and lose fat around the mid-section. They fall for these extreme fad diets out here that are so over-the-top with difficult protocols that no one can stick to for very long. You will attempt drastic measures, like massive calorie restriction, but then you end up binge eating after a few days because the diet is too drastic to maintain and you become too hungry.

The problem isn't with you or your willpower. The problem is with the approach you take. Getting healthy is a lifestyle change. It is something that you can incorporate day-in and day-out for the rest of your life. It is not something you do for two weeks, four weeks, two months, or one year. If you take the old and failing approach that you try each and every year (or multiple times a year in many cases), you take drastic measures for two weeks, you begin to see some results, and

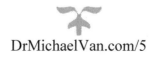

DrMichaelVan.com/5

then you stop. It is like you begin to get to your goal, but right when you start seeing the light at the end of the tunnel, you suddenly tank it and give up. You put in tons and tons of effort, you expend a tremendous amount of will power, you start seeing real positive changes, and then boom! You quit. This failed system is avoided with a balanced approach without extremes. An approach that is implemented as a long-term lifestyle change.

Here is my point. Why do we make these cosmetic type of goals? Instead of wanting to lose twenty pounds, why don't we just make our goal health and only health? Does a healthy person have excess fat in the midsection? Is a healthy person overweight? Does a healthy person have a minimal amount of lean muscle mass? Of course not. So let's just get healthy. The cool thing about health is that there is no endpoint. It is a daily decision for the rest of your life. If you put in the effort to achieve the state of health, then you will have the body you have always imagined having. You will have the physique and the small waist you have always dreamed about. You will have that low body fat and that healthy muscle mass you never thought would be possible. You will allow your body to function optimally and prevent chronic disease. You will be healthy and have all the benefits health comes with.

What I want to get across in this book is the fact that you can implement some simple steps on a consistent basis throughout your life and get life-changing results. If you were looking for a short-term special fad diet that takes tons of willpower, then this is the wrong book for you. However, if you want to incorporate a lifestyle change that is very doable and can help you towards the path of health, then this book is exactly what you have been missing.

CHAPTER 1:

COMMON PRACTICE OF TODAY:

SCIENCE OR PROPOGANDA?

We have all heard of the following facts….wait. We have all heard of the following theories we have regarded as facts:

- Cracking your knuckles causes arthritis

- The world is flat

- Deoxygenated blood is blue

- Once you lose brain cells, they are gone permanently

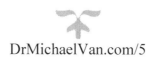

DrMichaelVan.com/5

- Breakfast is the most important meal of the day

- Eat many small meals throughout the day instead of a few large meals to keep metabolism high

The fact is, all those above statements are absolutely false with no research supporting these claims.

- Cracking your knuckles absolutely does not cause arthritis, and has never been shown to do so

- The world is round

- Deoxygenated blood is red (even though veins are blue in color)

Now let's move on to the last three theories regarding the loss of brain cells, breakfast, and multiple meals throughout the day. For many years, the medical field held the belief that the brain did not make major changes after a certain point in time. They believed the brain was 'fixed' or set on a specific path. They thought that once you lost brain cells, regardless of how you lost them, that the consequences were permanent. They thought the brain was static. The old belief was that a loss of brain cells as we age (or from a destructive lifestyle) was permanent, and there was nothing you could do about it. We now know the brain is able to change and develop in miraculous ways we never thought possible. In fact, our brain has the ability to regenerate and produce new cells throughout our lifetime in a process called neuroplasticity. Therefore, we can throw the brain cell myth we believed for hundreds of years out the window.

"But Tony the Tiger and the Quaker oatmeal man himself tell us that breakfast is the most important meal of the day!" Nutritionists will tell you to make sure you start your day with a healthy breakfast, so you can get that metabolism firing first thing in the morning to help you stay lean and thin. This idea has become so commonplace and mainstream that it is accepted as fact. Even today's official nutrition guidelines recommend that we eat breakfast. But what sort of research did they base these recommendations off of? Did it ever occur to you that the idea of breakfast being so important came directly from the manufacturers of breakfast food companies? Like Tony the Tiger of Frosted Flakes. Like Raisin Bran. Like Quaker Oatmeal. In fact, on the Quaker Oatmeal's very own website, it says that in 1882, the first national magazine advertising program for the importance of breakfast cereal was launched. I wonder how much science and research they used to back up that claim? How about none.

In fact, this matter was recently settled in a randomized controlled trial, the gold standard of science, in 2014. Experts compared the effects of eating breakfast and skipping breakfast on overall weight in 283 overweight adults. After 16 weeks, there was no statistically significant difference in weight loss between the two groups. This study out of *The American Journal of Clinical Nutrition* concludes that:

> *"Contrary to widely espoused views this had no discernable effect on weight loss in free-living adults who were attempting to lose weight."*

It turns out that for healthy adults, breakfast is actually not the most important meal of the day after all.

Did you know that if you went to a nutritionist for diet advice, they would no doubt tell you to eat six small meals a day so you can keep your metabolism high and avoid hitting the metabolic plateau known as 'starvation mode?' According to their claims, not eating makes your body think that it is starving, so it shuts down its metabolism and prevents you from burning fat. They even teach this concept at schools. Their theory is that if you eat small meals all day long, you allow your body to constantly burn extra calories and will allow your metabolism to fire at optimal capacity.

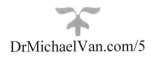

What if I were to tell you that there has never been one research article implementing small meals throughout the day, even though nearly every person has heard this recommendation and many implement it. Again, their claim to fame was that this type of eating regimen helped keep the body out of 'starvation mode.' They say that if you spread out 2000 calories into small meals throughout the day, you will burn more calories from the boost in metabolism compared to eating just two or three large meals. The theory of keeping metabolism high by always eating sounds good in principle, but in reality it is just that…a theory.

So what does the science say? Well, the actual literature tells a completely different story. It's true that your body does indeed have to burn extra calories to process meals. However, eating many small meals throughout the day to keep your metabolism up is a complete myth. What researchers found is that whether you eat 2000 calories in one meal or spread it out throughout the day, your body will burn the same number of calories processing and metabolizing the food. You heard that right. Consuming the same number of calories in two meals versus seven meals show no difference in calories burned between the two groups. In fact, there has never been a study showing that eating many small meals throughout the day resulted in weight loss. If anything, the abundance of calories you are consuming while eating many meals actually had the opposite effect. Wow! How did we fall for that hoax and how on earth do nutritionists and other people of authority continue to use, teach, and promote this theory that has been invalidated?

Let's take it a step further. There has actually been research on the 'starvation mode' theory, and this is what they found. It turns out that this 'starvation mode,' where your metabolism begins to tank, actually does exist. The problem? Instead of it occurring after two to three hours after a meal that many people still believe to this day, it actually occurs 72-96 hours after a meal. That is three to four days after a meal, not a few hours!

What was interesting is that your metabolic rate is actually INCREASED short term after fasting. In fact, studies conducted right after a fasting period have shown a metabolic rate increase of 3.6% - 14% for up to 48 hours. This is because the body will actually release the stress hormones adrenaline and noradrenaline (epinephrine and norepinephrine) to help sharpen the mind and give us energy. These hormones tell your fat cells to break down body fat and stimulate your metabolism. Think back to what it must have been like for humans in the hunter-gatherer days. These desirable traits of mind enhancement and energy would allow them to affectively search for food and kill prey, increasing survival. With that said, after several days of not

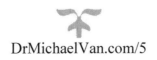

DrMichaelVan.com/5

eating, these intelligent adaptations would do more harm than good. We would not want our bodies to sustain a high metabolism and keep burning fuel three to four days after eating for fear of starvation. Therefore, our body will halt the increase in metabolism and the stress response after three to four days to conserve our energy and to increase the likelihood of survival.

The fact of the matter is that our body was built for periodic cycles of feast and famine. This mimics the eating habits of our ancestors. The evolutionary explanation for this is humans and other animals have fasted intermittently for much of their time on Earth. As a recent paper in the Proceedings of the National Academy of Sciences notes, "The most common eating pattern in modern societies, three meals plus snacks every day, is abnormal from an evolutionary perspective."

Our ancestors did not have access to grocery stores or food around the clock. There wasn't an Albertson's across the street next to a Taco Bell, which is a block away from a KFC and an In-N-Out Burger. They would cycle through periods of feast and famine, and this cycling produces a number of biochemical benefits that dramatically alters how your body operates. By imitating our ancestors and the conditions of cyclical nutrition, your body enters into a state of optimal functioning.

Our body simply cannot run properly when we are continuously fed. This is why eating all day triggers disease. Research shows that many biological repair and rejuvenation processes take place when there is an absence of food. Eating all day never allows your body the time to clean out all the garbage and regenerate.

Here is a quick breakdown of why multiple meals throughout the day is not healthy from a physiological perspective. When you eat a meal, your body spends a few hours processing that food and giving you readily available, easy to burn energy in its blood stream. Your body stores this easily available energy in the form of glycogen located in the muscle and liver. It uses this and your blood sugar as its first energy source because it is available. Sugar in the form of blood glucose and stored sugar in the form of glycogen are by far the body's preferred energy source before anything else.

Once those energy stores are used up, your body will then turn to its fat stores for energy. If you are constantly replenishing your glycogen stores and blood sugar by eating six small meals a day, how will your body ever be able to tap into its fat stores? It won't! The reason why so many struggle with their weight is because people rarely, if ever, skip a meal. As a result, they are adapted to burning sugar as their primary fuel, which will down-regulate enzymes that utilize and

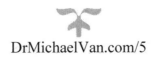

burn stored fat. In order to start using your fat stores as fuel

burning), your body has to be completely devoid of its blood sugar and

glycogen stores. This only happens when we go without food for a

period of eight to twelve hours. It only happens when we adopt the

eating pattern of our ancestors and put ourselves through periodic cycles

of feast and famine. It turns out our ancestors were right all along. *How*

surprising.

CHAPTER 2:

THE CASE FOR FASTING

Intermittent fasting is a phenomenon that is currently one of the world's most popular health and fitness trends. It involves alternating cycles of fasting and eating, instead of eating all hours during the day. It isn't a diet, but rather an eating pattern. It does not include any rules about what foods to eat, but rather when you should eat them.

As noted by Time magazine, intermittent fasting is becoming so popular because of one reason – it works. It works whether you are trying to lose weight, or just improve your biomarkers to achieve optimal health. In a nutshell, it is the way we are designed to eat. It allows us to use fat as our primary fuel instead of carbohydrates by adopting the way our ancestors used to eat.

THE SCIENTIFIC APPROACH TO
INTERMITTENT FASTING

Unlike so many diets out there, this is not the latest 'fad diet' portrayed in popular media. Dieting is a multi-billion dollar global industry, and there is not a shred of evidence people are becoming slimmer as a result. In fact, the opposite is true. The percentage of obesity keeps increasing and has now reached epidemic proportions all over the world. Statistics from 2012 show that over 35% of adults are obese, and 69% of adults are overweight. In 2014, the obesity rate among American adults hit 38%, a 3% increase in two years. A new study published by the *Lancet Medical Journal* found that for the first time in history, obese people now outnumber those who are underweight. In 2014, 641 million people were obese, compared to 105 million in 1975. Finally, by 2025, an estimated 20% of the global population and nearly half of American adults will be obese. That is just scary.

Losing weight is a big business worldwide. Weight loss programs, products, and other weight loss therapies generate more than $150 billion in profits in the US and Europe combined. By 2019, they estimate that the weight loss market will reach $206 billion. One study found that the average cost to lose roughly 11 lbs ranged from $755 for the Weight Watchers program to $2,730 for the weight loss medication Orlistat. Unfortunately, the end result for the majority of people on these diets is they end up spending thousands of dollars pursuing weight loss without any long-term success.

Studies show that the success rate of these diets for achieving long-term weight loss are extremely disappointing. One study looked at participants three years after they concluded a weight loss program. Only 12% kept off at least 75% of the weight they lost and 40% gained back more weight than they had originally lost. Think about that. You are almost four times as likely to put on more than your original starting weight than to actually lose weight long term. On top of all that, people actually pay for these horrific results!

Another study found that five years after a group of women lost weight during a six month weight loss program, they ended up gaining on average an additional 7.9 lbs more than their original starting weight. Yet another study found that only 19% of people on a weight loss diet were able to keep off 10% of the weight they lost in a five year period. This is the bottom line. Although a small percentage of people manage to lose weight and keep it off, most people regain all or a portion of the weight they lost, and many gain back even more weight.

A large factor that causes people on these weight loss programs to fail is an increase in appetite hormones that occurs when the body

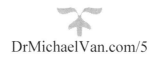

senses it has lost fat and muscle. Furthermore, calorie restriction and loss of muscle mass cause your body's metabolism to tank, making it easier to regain weight once you start eating normally again. Rather than producing lasting weight loss, dieting among non-obese people increases the risk of weight gain and obesity over time. There has got to be a better way out there.

Intermittent fasting, however, has proven to be a safe and effective approach that promotes not just fat loss, but actually improves overall health in ways no other lifestyle modification could do. What differentiates intermittent fasting from any other diet is the extreme abundance of high-quality, peer-reviewed research to back up all of its claims and results. It also serves as the way humans were physiologically designed to eat, period.

To have an effective long-term dietary and lifestyle intervention with sustained beneficial effects on metabolic and disease markers, there needs to be a strategy that promotes long-term adherence. These dietary interventions need to be palatable and satiating, meet minimal nutritional requirements, promote fat loss and the preservation of lean body mass, and ensure long-term safety. In addition, they also need to be simple to apply and monitor, and have widespread public health utility. Intermittent fasting achieves all this criteria and then some.

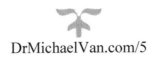

Dr. Stephen Freedland, a professor of urology and pathology at Duke University Medical Center, revealed how fasting was the only experimental approach out there that consistently improved survival rates in animals with cancer, as well as extended overall lifespan by as much as 30%.

A study published in the *International Journal of Obesity* found that intermittent fasting was just as effective as continuous fasting for weight loss and improving metabolic disease markers for obesity and chronic disease. These metabolic disease markers include total and LDL cholesterol, blood pressure, C-reactive protein, sex hormone binding globulin, IGF binding proteins, leptin, and free androgen index. The fact that intermittent fasting provides nearly identical health benefits as traditional continuous fasting is a very good thing because it is a lot easier to implement.

In addition, intermittent fasting was actually more effective than continuous fasting in perhaps the most important marker for health, which is reducing insulin resistance. Those of you who are unfamiliar with insulin resistance, it is a pathological condition in which cells fail to respond to the normal actions of the hormone insulin. Insulin resistance leads to nearly every chronic disease out there, including type II diabetes, heart disease, cancer, and stroke. More on insulin will be discussed later in Chapter 8.

Mark Mattson, a senior investigator for the National Institute on Aging, which is part of the US National Institute of Health (NIH), came up with the explanation on why intermittent fasting works:

> *"During the fasting period, cells are under a mild stress, and they respond to the stress adaptively by enhancing their ability to cope with stress and, maybe, to resist disease... There is considerable similarity between how cells respond to the stress of exercise and how cells respond to intermittent fasting."*

This is amazing news! We have long known that continuous fasting offers tons of health benefits, but realistically, who is going to do this? Who is going to go multiple days of intense caloric restriction to obtain these benefits? I know I wouldn't. What makes intermittent fasting so appealing is that it provides nearly identical health benefits (and superior benefits in some categories) without being so difficult to implement and maintain.

In a 2007 study out of the *American Journal of Clinical Nutrition,* researchers divided study participants into two groups. Each

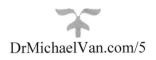

group consumed the same number of calories. The only difference was that one group consumed all their calories in three meals spread out throughout the day, while the other practiced intermittent fasting, consuming the same number of calories but in a restricted time frame. What they discovered was astonishing. The participants who ate in a smaller window of time had a significant improvement in body composition, including a substantial reduction in fat mass.

Another very interesting study looked at Muslim individuals following Ramadan. Ramadan is a holy month in the Islamic calendar, where Muslims must abstain from eating or drinking during daylight hours. This equates to approximately 12 hours of fasting each day. This study gave us one of the more natural models to study the intermittent fasting effects in humans. Aksungar, the author of this study, evaluated cardiovascular health in Muslim individuals before and after the completion of Ramadan.

The results showed significant improvements in their lipid profile and cholesterol levels, decreasing their overall risk of heart disease. Their blood was also healthier and they experienced an improved blood coagulation profile. This means that the body was less likely to form inappropriate blood clots, preventing stroke and blockages in the arteries. This study of Ramadan also exhibited a major decrease in harmful inflammation levels.

Again, intermittent fasting is not a diet. It is a pattern of eating. It is simply a way of scheduling your meals throughout the day so you can get the most out of them. Intermittent fasting is not about changing what and how much you eat. Instead, it is focused on changing when you eat. It is an easy way to get lean and meet your health goals without the crazy calorie-cutting diets.

What makes intermittent fasting so simple is it requires very little behavioral change. It falls into the category where it is simple enough to actually do it, but meaningful enough that it will make a huge difference. It is much easier for people to restrict their eating to a narrow window of time each day than to dramatically decrease their overall daily caloric intake.

I am particularly fond of the concepts of simplifying tasks, reducing stress, and being very efficient with my time. Intermittent fasting provides this simplicity to my life. I don't have to wake up in the morning and think about what to make for breakfast. I just brew my organic black coffee and I am off to work. Intermittent fasting allows me to eat one less meal each day, which means I get to plan one less

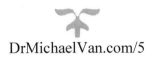

meal and cook one less meal each day. The simplicity is the best reason to give it a try. It provides countless health benefits without requiring massive behavioral and lifestyle change.

I truly believe this is the most powerful intervention out there if you're struggling with your health, weight, or any chronic disease. In addition, the other benefits it has to offer are nothing short of spectacular.

The list of health benefits includes, but are not limited to:

1. Massive fat burning and weight loss
2. Increased human growth hormone production
3. Enhanced brain function
4. Insulin sensitivity
5. Improvement of beneficial gut bacteria
6. Reduction in cancer
7. Leptin sensitivity
8. Ghrelin hormone normalization (hunger hormone)
9. Elimination of sugar cravings
10. Reduced oxidative stress
11. Increased lifespan and longevity

In this book we will go over the many benefits intermittent fasting can bring to you. It is also going to cover the specific ways you can implement this fasting regimen in your life, as well as going over common questions and concerns you might have. The scientific health benefits we go over are very important. A lot of these benefits will seem exaggerated, but this is simply a review of the scientific literature and is not mere opinion on my part.

If you don't want to know all the science that validates intermittent fasting as one of the most effective lifestyle changes you can do to increase health on all levels, then feel free to skip ahead to the chapters at the end. These chapters will go over specific plans of intermittent fasting you can choose from, as well as how to specifically implement each one.

With that said, I highly recommend you read through the whole book. From experience, when you know the benefits to something first, it makes implementation a lot easier. When you know the numerous benefits of fasting, it gives us a big "WHY" before we begin this journey. Once you know why we should implement intermittent fasting to our daily regimen, it becomes a lot easier to implement. No one would exercise if you didn't know the benefits of exercise on our health. No one would eat healthy foods that you do not at least enjoy if you

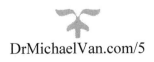

didn't know it was necessary to live a long healthy life. That goes without saying. If you have a big enough 'why,' you will figure out the 'how.'

CHAPTER 3:

FAT BURNING

Weight loss and fat loss is perhaps the most common reason people try intermittent fasting in the first place. With the increasing obesity epidemic going on around the world, there has been a widespread search for an effective dietary approach to aid in weight and fat loss. Unlike so many diets out there, this is a safe and effective approach that promotes not just fat loss, but has an extreme abundance of research to back it up.

This worldwide obesity epidemic creates a strong need for an effective new weight loss approach that can:

1. Prevent weight gain

2. Promote fat and weight loss

3. Maintain a healthy weight once ideal weight is reached

With over half of the population in the United States, United Kingdom, and many other developed countries being collectively overweight or obese, there is tons of pressure to achieve these goals from both a public health and a clinical perspective.

Like I briefly mentioned before, when your body expends energy, it first grabs its energy stores from your available blood sugar and your glycogen stores. It takes on average about 8-12 hours for your body to metabolize and use up all its blood sugar and glycogen stores after a meal is consumed. After you use up these energy stores, then your body will start to make a shift to burning fat for energy. What this means is that your body will only tap into its fat stores and start to burn fat as energy when 8-12 hours have passed after a meal is consumed.

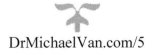

DrMichaelVan.com/5

Figure 3.1: Order of Energy Usage

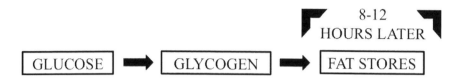

When you apply intermittent fasting and shift your body into an efficient fat-burning machine, your cravings for unhealthy foods and carbs will automatically disappear! This is because your body is now able to burn your stored fat as energy instead of being dependent on fast-burning carbs for fuel. Fat, being the slow-burning fuel that it is, allows you to keep your energy levels high without suffering from the dramatic energy crash that is associated with sugar. If you are not hungry, then guess what? Not eating for several hours becomes no big deal. You don't have to have extreme willpower or enormous levels of self-discipline to maintain this eating schedule. This makes it much easier to maintain a healthy body weight you have always desired.

The science validates this time and time again. The New York Times recently reported on a recent 38-week study out of the journal *Cell Metabolism* analyzing the effect different eating schedules had on the health of male mice. Half of the mice were allowed to eat whenever they wanted, while the other half only had access to food during a restricted period of time. At the end of the 38 weeks, the mice that were allowed to eat during all hours of the day became obese and suffered with metabolic dysfunctions. The mice that were restricted to eating within a specific time window remained thin and healthy. This was in spite of both groups eating the exact same food and consuming the same amount of calories.

Intermittent fasting prevents obesity from ever occurring, and this premise still held true even without any type of calorie restriction. What this means is that mice could eat anything they wanted during their eating window and still remain lean and fit throughout life. This study also showed the exact same findings in human subjects.

Figure 3.2: Prevention of Obesity

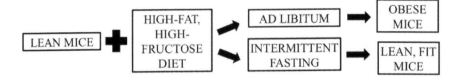

This conclusion also held true even when the restricted group of mice were allowed to cheat on weekends, eating at any time they wanted! In fact, they were still able to get many of the protective effects fasting provides. This is particularly relevant to the modern human lifestyle. After all, many people do like to splurge and have 'cheat days' during the weekends by going out to eat and consume an occasional alcoholic beverage.

Figure 3.3: The Effects of 'Cheat Days'

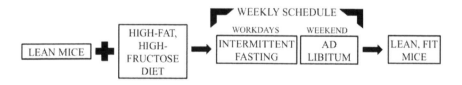

Finally, this study tested intermittent fasting's ability to be a therapeutic intervention against those already with obesity. Currently, treatment for obesity is very limited and many models only offer modest improvements at best. What they found was astonishing. Intermittent fasting not only prevented obesity, but it also reversed the harmful effects of obesity caused by chronic unhealthy diets. It stabilized and reversed the progression of metabolic diseases in mice with preexisting obesity and other metabolic disorders, including type II diabetes, fatty liver, and high cholesterol.

Figure 3.4: Reversal of Metabolic Dysfunction

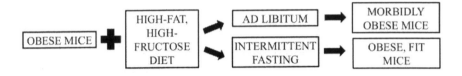

If you utilize the nutrition protocols of small meals throughout the day, you are constantly replenishing your blood sugar and glycogen stores. Therefore, you will never allow your body to shift to fat burning mode. I wonder why people utilizing that eating technique never got the results they expected and lost the fat they always wanted? (Sarcasm) The reason why many struggle with their weight is because they're in continuous feast mode and rarely, if ever, go without a meal. Their bodies become adapted to only burning sugar as its primary fuel, which in turn down-regulates the enzymes that utilize and burn stored fat.

In contrast, when your body is in a fasted state of more than eight to twelve hours after your last meal, your body doesn't have a recently consumed meal to use as energy. It forces your body to pull energy from the fat stored in your body. Again, this is because there is no available glucose in your blood stream or glycogen in your muscles and liver.

This is one of the main reasons why many patients of mine have lost a tremendous amount of fat without changing what they eat, how much they eat, or how often they exercise. Intermittent fasting puts your body in the fat burning state that you rarely make it to during a normal eating schedule. Don't get me wrong, it is absolutely critical to eat healthy foods, because at the end of the day, you are what you eat. The point here is that you can get fat burning results without changing anything but the timing of your meals.

Based on my research and my very own experience, intermittent fasting is the most powerful way to shift your body into fat burning mode. This is the same concept when you exercise in a fasted state. Exercising after you have been fasting for at least a period of 8-16 hours dramatically increases fat burning. Without the glucose and glycogen to pull energy from during your workout, your body is forced to adapt and pull its energy from fat. Since your metabolic demand during a workout is way higher than at rest, you will be burning way more fat during your workout. This leads to a much more efficient and effective workout giving you amazing fat burning results! More information regarding how to maximize your workout will be discussed in my next book.

Figure 3.5: Fasted State Exercise

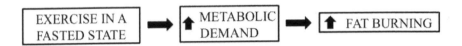

In terms of weight loss, intermittent fasting has shown to be a very powerful way to shed those unwanted pounds. In a study review from 2014, it was shown to cause weight loss of 3-8% over periods of 3-24 weeks. That is a very large amount compared to most weight loss studies. In addition, people also lost 4-7% of their waist circumference during the same duration. Lowering waist circumference means that people lost significant amounts of the harmful belly fat that builds up around your organs and causes disease. Since this diet is extremely safe, easy to comply with, and promotes long-term adherence, it serves as the most effective weight loss strategy around.

Another reason (although not required) intermittent fasting can work so well for weight loss is that it helps you eat fewer calories. If for example, you skip breakfast every day and only consume food between the hours of 12-8pm, you are essentially skipping a whole meal. Unless you completely compensate by eating much more during your eating period, then you will no doubt be taking in fewer calories. Calorie counting here is not required, because it makes it so much easier to eat less when you have to skip a meal. It is a convenient way to restrict calories without consciously trying to eat less.

Intermittent fasting also causes less muscle loss than the more traditional approaches to weight loss, such as continuous calorie restriction. One of the worst side effects of traditional dieting is that your body tends to burn lean healthy muscle in the process instead of the fat that most people are seeking to lose. According to a study out of the journal *Obesity Reviews*, intermittent fasting causes much less muscle loss than the standard methods of weight loss, giving intermittent fasting superior benefits in preserving lean body mass.

Figure 3.6: Fasting and Muscle Loss

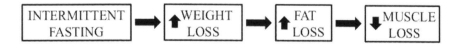

When you lose weight by reducing the amount of calories you eat (continuous calorie restriction), approximately 75% of that weight is lost as fat mass, and roughly 25% is lost as fat free mass (or muscle).

Figure 3.7: Continuous Calorie Restriction and Muscle Loss

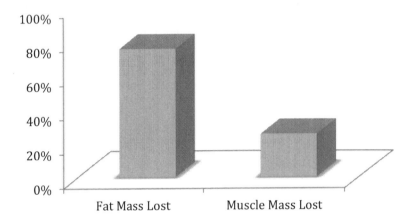

With intermittent fasting, a much lower proportion of muscle mass is lost. On average, around 90% of the weight loss was lost in the form of fat, and only 10% of the weight loss was lost in the form of muscle. That is a huge difference! 25% muscle loss on the standard diet of continuous calorie restriction compared to only 10% muscle loss in the intermittent fasting based regimens.

Figure 3.7: Intermittent Fasting and Muscle Loss

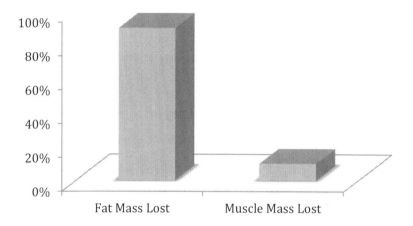

The amount of muscle or fat free mass in the body is the main predictor of your basal metabolic rate. Basal metabolic rate (BMR) is the amount of energy your body expends while at rest. It is basically how many calories your body burns when you are not doing any activity. The more muscle you have, the higher your metabolism will be. The more muscle you lose, the lower your metabolism will be.

THE SCIENTIFIC APPROACH TO
INTERMITTENT FASTING

The strong evidence highlighting how intermittent fasting can help you hold on to more muscle mass compared to standard calorie restriction cannot be denied. Not only is having a greater amount of lean muscle mass more aesthetically pleasing to the eye, but it also results in a higher metabolic rate. The higher your metabolism, the more you will continue to keep your body in a fat burning state.

It is wise to choose dietary interventions that preserve as much lean muscle mass as possible in order to take advantage of the increase in metabolism and physique. That cannot be understated here. You literally have the potential to get shredded and extremely cut by doing intermittent fasting and going on an exercise program. You will keep muscle mass at its peak while keeping fat down to a minimum. If you always wanted that amazing body of your dreams, stop wishing it could happen and just apply this stuff. If it worked for me and countless others, it can work for you!

A couple things to consider regarding these values is this is for the average study participant under 'normal' conditions. These values of 75% fat / 25% muscle and 90% fat / 10% muscle assumes no exercise. What we do know is that exercise helps preserve muscle mass. Therefore, you may actually see the percent of muscle loss actually decrease slightly from the values reported in both the intermittent fasting

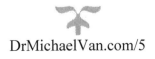

DrMichaelVan.com/5

and the continuous calorie restriction categories. The net effect, however, would still be the same and reign strongly in favor of intermittent fasting. In addition, proper protein intake after exercise will help improve muscle retention during any weight loss regimen because of its muscle-sparing effect. Again, this would benefit both groups so intermittent fasting is still far superior.

There are several ways intermittent fasting causes massive fat burning in the body. Not only does it force your body to attack its fat stores, but it actually changes the activity of your hormones in order to facilitate fat loss. Insulin is a hormone produced in the pancreas that is released when we eat. When we fast, insulin levels decrease dramatically, which facilitates fat burning. Levels of growth hormone skyrocket during your fasting period, leading to fat loss and muscle gain. Norepinephrine levels (noradrenaline) are also increased in the body in response to fasting. Your nervous system sends norepinephrine to your fat cells, stimulating the breakdown of body fat into free fatty acids that can be burned for energy during your fast. Together, these hormonal changes promote the loss of body weight and belly fat.

Figure 3.8: Intermittent Fasting and Hormonal Changes

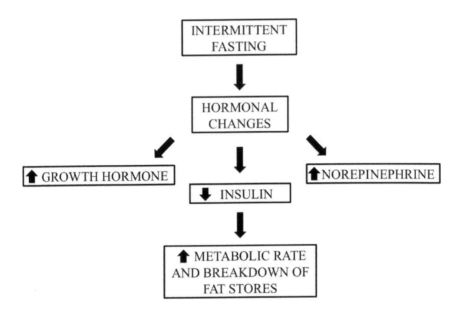

The take home message is clear. Intermittent fasting promotes massive fat loss. The lowering of insulin, increase in growth hormone, and the increase in norepinephrine (noradrenaline) adds to the amazing fat burning effect as well as the increase in metabolic rate. It leads to several physiological changes in the body that basically make fat burning a lot easier. With that being said, the benefits of intermittent fasting go way beyond fat and weight loss as you will see. It provides numerous benefits to your metabolic health, immune system, gut microbiome, and your lifespan.

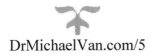

CHAPTER 4:

GROWTH HORMONE PRODUCTION

Human growth hormone, or HGH, is a hormone that is made by the pituitary gland and released into the bloodstream. The pituitary releases HGH in bursts; levels rise following exercise, trauma, and sleep. Under normal conditions, more HGH is produced at night than during the day because of the indirect relationship it has with insulin. HGH levels rise during childhood, peaks during puberty, and declines from middle age onward.

What is interesting is the relationship between growth hormone and the hormone insulin. When you consume food, your body responds with insulin production. Insulin is a hormone that basically transports blood glucose (sugar) from a recently consumed meal into the cells of your body. It allows your cells to take in blood sugar for energy or storage, depending on what is needed at the time. The more sensitive you are to insulin, the more likely you will be using the food you consume efficiently.

It turns out that the more sensitive you are to insulin, the more growth hormone you will secrete. They have an indirect relationship, meaning as insulin levels increase, human growth hormone secretion decreases and vice versa. HGH is only released when there is no insulin released in the blood stream, and this only happens during a fasted state and when you are sleeping. For example, when you are sleeping, you are not eating, so there is no blood sugar from a recently consumed meal to signal your body to release insulin. This allows growth hormone levels to rise in response to the low levels of insulin during periods of sleep.

What researchers have found is that your body is most sensitive to insulin following a period of fasting. The reason being is simple; if you do the opposite and eat all day long, insulin is constantly being released. Eventually your body will become unresponsive to the constant release of insulin. It's kind of like hearing an annoying sound. At first, you are very responsive to the annoying sound and it is very irritating. Eventually, however, you start to adapt to the sound and it

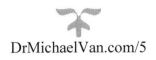

doesn't bother you anymore. It's the same thing that happens on airplanes to the sound of the engine, or when someone is constantly nagging at you. Eventually, you get used to the stimulus and don't react anymore.

According to the American College of Cardiology, fasting triggered a 1,300% increase in human growth hormone secretion in women, and an astounding 2,000% increase in men! This statistic alone is a definitive reason to drop what you're doing and incorporate intermittent fasting into your lifestyle immediately. HGH, commonly known as your fitness hormone, plays a huge role in your health, fitness, and longevity. It actively promotes muscle growth, and even further boosts fat loss by increasing your metabolism. The fact that it simultaneously aids in muscle building and fat loss explains how HGH can help you get lean and lose weight without sacrificing your beneficial muscle mass you've worked so hard for.

The advantages of HGH go much further than muscle building and fat loss. It also works in the body to increase:

- Healing, growth, and repair of essentially every tissue in the body, including bone
- Libido
- Protein synthesis
- Production of other anabolic hormones
- Immune system function
- Energy

This is why athletes who are already at a healthy weight can benefit greatly from intermittent fasting. The only intervention that can even come close in terms of dramatically increasing HGH levels is high-intensity interval training, which will be discussed in my next book. Why do you think so many professional sports organizations such as Major League Baseball and the National Football League are banning synthetic HGH? Because it greatly increases performance, muscle mass, and recovery! If only these athletes knew about the impact intermittent fasting and high-intensity interval training has on HGH. Increasing these levels by up to 2,000% (this percentage is actually greater if combined with high-intensity interval training) is absolutely a mind

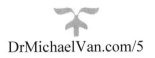

blowing statistic we can't ignore. In fact, this is something that even artificial injections can't accomplish.

Besides athletes, many other populations are starting to experiment in the illicit use of synthetic HGH injections for a variety of reasons. These include slowing down the aging process, the massive fat burning effect and the amazing muscle building capability. It's becoming a trend for more and more adults using HGH injections for anti-aging and longevity reasons. According to Harvard Medical School, many practitioners offer expensive injections of synthetic human growth hormone, even though the FDA has not approved the use of HGH for anti-aging, bodybuilding, or athletic enhancement. The marketing or distribution of the hormone for any of these purposes is illegal in the U.S. According to one estimate, 100,000 people received HGH without a valid prescription in 2002. According to a New York Post article in 2014, experimentation with human growth hormone by teenagers more than doubled in the past year. More and more of the younger population are looking to drugs to boost their athletic performance and improve their looks.

As with any hormone replacement therapy, the artificial hormones that are injected are never the exact same structure as the body's natural hormone. The term bio-identical is misleading in that aspect, as you can't duplicate in a lab what naturally occurs in your body. Therefore, this practice of synthetic injections comes with a high rate of harmful side effects, including fluid retention, joint pain, breast enlargement, carpal tunnel syndrome, diabetes, heart disease, and cancer (especially prostate cancer). As always, your best bet is to work on maximizing your body's natural ability to secrete HGH, which comes with no harmful side effects. The fact of the matter is that intermittent fasting (and high-intensity interval training) will allow you to experience all the positive benefits and increase your overall health at the same time.

Figure 4.1: Intermittent Fasting and Human Growth Hormone

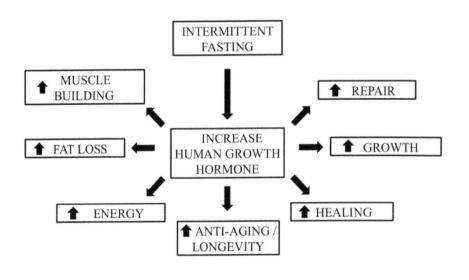

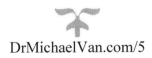

CHAPTER 5:

BRAIN FUNCTION

For many years, the medical field held firmly to the belief that the brain was fixed and static. It was thought that the brain was incapable of making major changes after a certain point in time, and that any loss of brain cells from destructive lifestyle habits had permanent consequences. Doctors rendered any degenerative brain disorder as irreversible with treatment options only consisting of symptom management as brain function slowly faded away.

We now know that the brain is a complex, dynamic structure. It is actually able to change and develop throughout our entire lifetime. It is plastic, malleable, pliable, flexible, and impressionable. Neuroplasticity is the term researchers now use to describe the brain's

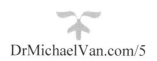

DrMichaelVan.com/5

dynamic ability to reorganize itself by forming new neural connections throughout life. Neuroplasticity allows nerve cells (neurons) to heal after injury or disease, as well as helping brain cells adapt to ever-changing situations and environments.

The brain can heal itself by a few different mechanisms. It can do something called axonal sprouting, where undamaged axons grow new nerve endings to reconnect cells whose links were injured. An axon, or nerve fiber, is a long projection of a nerve cell that typically conducts electrical impulses away from the neuron's cell body. The function of the axon is to transmit information to different nerve cells, muscles and glands. Undamaged axons can also spread out nerve endings and connect with other undamaged nerve cells, forming new pathways and connections in the brain. If one hemisphere of the brain is damaged or isn't functioning correctly, the intact hemisphere can take over some of its functions by using the ability to reorganize and form new connections between the intact neurons.

The nervous system consists of the brain, spinal cord, sensory organs, and all of the nerves that connect these organs with the rest of the body. In order for the nervous system to properly respond to environmental challenges, certain neurotrophic factors need to be present. Neurotrophic factors are a family of proteins that support the

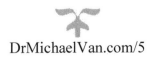

growth, survival, and differentiation of both developing and mature brain cells. These neurotrophic factors allow the body to go through a series of mechanisms that lead to the remodeling and the birth of new brain and nerve cells. In fact, researchers found a direct link between brain cell survival and the amounts of specific neurotrophic factors available.

Neurotrophic factors are also responsible for the construction and refinement of new brain connections that occur when these cells regenerate. They control growth and remodeling of axons, aid in the function of membrane receptors in the brain, help the brain release neurotransmitters and aid in the communication process between cells. This process of neuroplasticity and brain cell regeneration has the capability of lasting well into adulthood. The bottom line is this: Specific neurotrophic factors need to be present in order for neuroplasticity to take place.

Through various studies and research, the specific neurotrophic factor serving as the crucial mediator of neuroplasticity is called brain-derived neurotrophic factor, also known as BDNF. Interestingly enough, this special neurotrophic factor activates brain stem cells in order to increase the production of new brain cells. Remember when you've been told that once you lost brain cells, they were gone

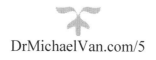

permanently? We now know that that statement is completely false

illustrated by the abundant recent research on neuroplasticity.

Brain and nerve cells need to be stimulated by specific activity in

order to produce BDNF, which is required for neuroplasticity to take

place in the brain. Put another way, BDNF serves as the bridge between

specific activity of the body and the regeneration and production of new

brain tissue.

If we know that BDNF is required for optimal brain functioning,

the question then becomes, what activity does this? What action

increases the production of BDNF? This is where intermittent fasting

enters the equation.

Intermittent fasting affects brain function by massively

increasing the production of this special protein. In fact, intermittent

fasting has been shown to increase BDNF by a factor of 50 to 400

percent, depending on the specific region of the brain we are dealing

with. BDNF is more abundant in areas of the brain that show the highest

capability of regeneration.

One such area that neuroplasticity occurs in the brain from

intermittent fasting is in the hippocampus. The hippocampus, located

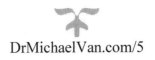

deep in the temporal lobes of the brain, deals with the formation of long-term memories and spatial navigation. The production of new brain cells in this area from intermittent fasting can lead to enhanced brain functioning in areas such as special learning, pattern discrimination, contextual memory and mood regulation.

Figure 5.1: Intermittent Fasting and BDNF

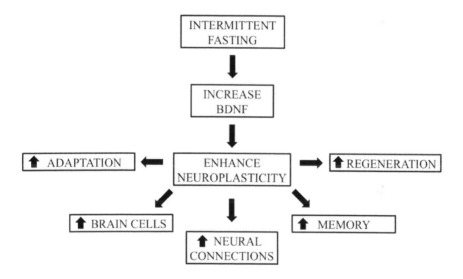

A recent article in the journal *Cell Metabolism* describes how intermittent fasting promotes neurogenesis of the hippocampus and improves cognitive performance in mice. Intermittent fasting literally produced multi-system regeneration of brain tissue. Immune and brain function significantly improved, lifespan was increased and the risk of inflammatory and metabolic diseases reduced significantly. In the mouse brain, neurons were regenerated, especially in the hippocampus. Together, this improved learning ability, memory and concentration. Researchers followed this study up by performing a human pilot study and found the exact same results on the improvement of brain function in humans.

Figure 5.2: Multi-System Regeneration

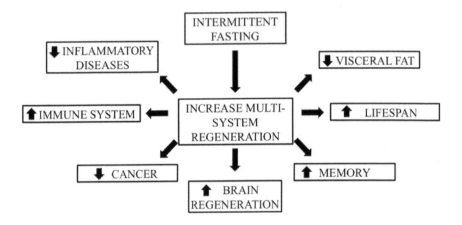

This multi-system regeneration also included reductions of visceral belly fat, the harmful fat surrounding organs, as well as the risk for cancer and inflammatory diseases. As if that wasn't enough, it also reduced the incidence of skin lesions and it ceased bone mineral density loss. Intermittent fasting actually allowed for healthy bone formation to take place, reversing osteoporosis.

It is clear that the hippocampus, as well as the rest of the brain, is positively influenced by intermittent fasting. What we also know is that the hippocampus is negatively stimulated by factors such as stress and inflammation. The consequences inflammation has on neurogenesis and neuroplasticity are profound. These include a decrease in the survival rate of neurons and the ability to make new neurons. It also has detrimental implications on cognition, resulting in a decline in memory and the ability to learn new things. For example, a potent marker of inflammation and stress called tumor necrosis factor—alpha (TNF-α), has been linked to a number of devastating effects on brain function. The presence of abnormal levels of TNF-α is associated with low quantities of neural stem cells, a decrease in the brain's ability to make new cells and more degenerative processes in the brain.

What is BDNF's role in degenerative brain disorders, such as Alzheimer's and Parkinson's disease, as well as clinical depression? It

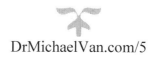

is now clear that many of these common brain disorders have been linked to critically low levels of BDNF. This special protein protects your brain cells from detrimental changes associated with these brain disorders. It accomplishes this by generating and recruiting other chemicals that aid in brain cell health.

Mark Mattson, a senior investigator for the National Institute on Aging, which is part of the US National Institute of Health (NIH), talks about a study on a population of mice engineered to develop Alzheimer's-like symptoms. He explains the effect intermittent fasting had on this population:

> *"Fasting begun in middle age delayed the onset of memory problems by about six months. This is a large effect, perhaps equivalent to 20 years in humans."*

When mice genetically engineered to develop Alzheimer's were put on an intermittent fasting regimen, they started to develop Alzheimer's symptoms around the age of two. In human terms, that is the equivalent to being ninety years of age. Normally, the mice would develop the symptoms of dementia in half that time, or around one year of age. That is equivalent to forty or fifty years of age in humans. This means that there is a potential delay of dementia-like symptoms in

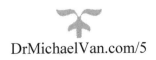

humans of up to forty to fifty years! Furthermore, when these mice in the study were put on a junk food diet and were able to eat freely throughout the day, they started to develop dementia in as little as nine months! This suggests that the severity and occurrence of such horrible symptoms of dementia are directly linked to lifestyle factors, specifically the way you eat and what you eat.

Wow, pretty profound statement there. You probably know family members, or have friends that have family members, who have been affected by Alzheimer's disease. It is terrible. Victims of this disease lose the ability to remember almost anything, including the names of their own kids. Imagine being able to possibly delay the progression of memory loss by twenty to fifty years. Do you think that would make a huge difference to families worldwide?

BDNF also has benefits in regards to protecting your neuro-muscular system from degradation. This is accomplished by BDNF's effect on the neuro-motors of the body, the specific site where the nervous system communicates with the muscular system. It is where the nerve sends signals to your muscles to do work and contract. Without it, nothing would happen and you would not be able to produce any movement. Think of it from this analogy. Your muscular system is your engine, and your neuro-motor is the ignition. Without a well-functioning neuro-motor, your muscle would be like an engine without ignition.

By the way, neuro-motor degradation is why there is a decrease in muscle mass as you age. By restoring optimal BDNF levels from intermittent fasting, you will benefit both your muscles and your brain. This muscle and brain connection is a big reason why exercise has such a large impact on your brain function. This is yet another reason why the combination of intermittent fasting and high intensity interval training can exponentially magnify your results.

As if that wasn't enough, in a study out of *The Journal of Nutritional Biochemistry*, Mattson compared the benefits of intermittent fasting (IF) and caloric restriction (CR) to that of physical exercise. He states the following:

> *"Recent findings suggest that some of the beneficial effects of IF on both the cardiovascular system and the brain are mediated by brain-derived neurotrophic factor signaling in the brain. Interestingly, cellular and molecular effects of IF and CR on the cardiovascular system and the brain are similar to those of regular physical exercise, suggesting shared mechanisms."*

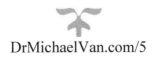

We all know that exercise provides tons of physiological benefits to the human body. In fact, it is the only other lifestyle factor besides fasting that has been shown to increase the production of BDNF. With that said, certain types of exercise programs prove far superior to others when it comes to BDNF production. It is wise to choose a program that involves high-intensity interval training to maximize this potential, which will be discussed in my next book.

Movement of the spine and other joints of the body stimulate brain activity by sending massive sensory input to the brain. This is why when you exercise, you feel like you can concentrate better due to the fact that your brain has been immensely stimulated by the movement. This is also why when you don't move all day, you feel sluggish and tired as if you had brain fog. Even though you spent all day conserving all of your energy, you still feel sluggish because your brain wasn't getting proper stimulation from movement. The fact that they can relate the benefits of physical exercise to the benefits of intermittent fasting is very promising.

Besides the amazing benefits an increase in BDNF levels have on brain function, intermittent fasting also benefits your brain by using fat as a primary fuel. In fact, burning fat as the main fuel of your body helps the enhancement of your brain performance by further preserving your memory and learning ability. Let me explain.

When you are roughly eight hours into your fast, your body then starts to utilize its fat stores for energy. This only occurs once your body is depleted of glucose and glycogen, which again takes around eight to twelve hours. This process involves the breakdown of fatty acids by your liver to form ketone bodies. These ketone bodies are then released into the bloodstream and used up by your body for energy. In fact, ketones are actually the preferred fuel for the majority of your brain instead of glucose. Utilizing ketones for energy provides protective benefits to neurons, also known as your brain cells. When we allow our brain to get the majority of its fuel from ketone bodies instead of glucose, we get improvements in memory and learning. This energy source also helps slow disease processes down in the brain, again preventing such disorders as Alzheimer's.

In summary, intermittent fasting holds the key for enhanced brain functioning. It also has very promising evidence on preventing brain degenerative disorders, such as Alzheimer's and Parkinson's disease. If you are suffering from memory loss, if you feel as though you are always in a state of 'brain fog,' or better yet, you just want to maximize the potential of your brain function, implement intermittent

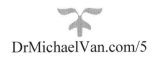

fasting immediately. By eating the way you were designed to, you will no doubt get the protective brain benefits you have always desired.

CHAPTER 6:

INCREASE LIFESPAN AND LONGEVITY

Who wants to live a longer, happier, healthier life with tons of energy and vitality? Who wants to be active and robust until your 80's and late 90's? Who wants to reverse and prevent signs and biomarkers of aging with scientifically proven methods throughout your entire lifespan? These are proven methods that not only reverse and slow down the aging process, but also protect and restore healthy brain and immune function, growth hormone production, fat loss, lean muscle mass, and insulin sensitivity. Additionally, these proven methods significantly lower your risk of diabetes, cardiovascular disease, blood pressure, inflammation, and cancer. Anyone interested?

This is exactly what intermittent fasting does. Fasting has been scientifically proven to slow down the aging process, reduce age-related chronic diseases, and extend lifespan. This has been shown in a variety of species, including rats, fish, worms, and yeast. In some cases, restricting calories caused an increase in lifespan by as much as fifty percent! Since you operate under the same physiological principles of nature as other animals, there is evidence that fasting has a similar effect on human lifespan.

Scientists have figured out that cells in our body react to intermittent fasting in a similar fashion as they do to exercise. Fasting, like exercise, is a stressor to our system. When we place our bodies under a healthy type of stress, regardless if it is in the form of exercise or fasting, we create changes at the cellular level that enable us to extend our lifespan.

Mark Mattson, the senior investigator for the National Institute on Aging, explained the concept of intermittent fasting and how it relates to stress:

> *"During the fasting period, cells are under a mild stress, and they respond to the stress adaptively by enhancing their ability to cope with stress and, maybe, to resist disease… There is*

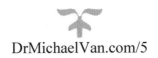

DrMichaelVan.com/5

considerable similarity between how cells respond to the stress of exercise and how cells respond to intermittent fasting."

Furthermore, Mattson says in the study out of the journal *Ageing Research Reviews*, that "intermittent fasting increases lifespan and protects various tissues against disease, in part, by Hormesis mechanisms that increase cellular stress resistance." When our bodies are placed under a healthy form of stress like intermittent fasting, we enable our bodies to become stronger and respond to negative stressors in a more productive manner. It is similar to exercise. When we expose ourselves to the stress exercise provides, we are able to withstand more physical stress as a result. We build up tolerance to lower intensities of exercise, and are able to tolerate ever-increasing workloads as a result.

FAT VS CARBOHYDRATES:
FREE RADICALS

To really understand the potential that intermittent fasting has for increasing lifespan and longevity, we have to look at the physiological effects of transitioning our bodies from burning carbohydrates as fuel to burning fat as our primary fuel. Fat is a cleaner form of energy than carbohydrates and it improves insulin sensitivity. Burning fat also generates far less reactive oxygen species (ROS), also known as free radicals. Glucose is known as a more "dirty" type of fuel because it produces a lot more free radicals. Free radicals are responsible for cellular and DNA damage and are linked to an increased potential for illness and disease.

One way to combat this free radical damage is to consume an abundance of antioxidants that can provide an adequate defense against them. These antioxidants include glutathione, vitamin C, resveratrol, carotenoids, astaxanthin, CoQ10, alpha-lipoic acid, and vitamin E. This is why you often hear about the importance of antioxidants in your diet. Rich sources of antioxidants include blueberries, acai and several other raw fruits and vegetables. As long as you consume a balanced, unprocessed diet full of high-quality raw organic vegetables and fruits, your body will acquire these essential antioxidants naturally.

The best way to reduce these free radicals isn't necessarily to provide a good defense against them in the form of antioxidants (although that is important), but to avoid the excessive free radical damage in the first place. This happens when your body starts burning a clean fuel like fat instead of the dirty fuel consisting of an abundance of carbs. In addition, when your caloric intake is greater than necessary, or when you consume food at times when you have low energy needs, it increases the number of free radicals produced.

This is especially true when you eat immediately before you go to bed. You are building up fuel when it is not needed. This is why I recommend not eating at least a couple hours before bedtime. Your body uses the least amount of calories when sleeping, so the last thing you would want to do is consume an excess amount of calories during this time. This will generate an abundance of free radicals that can damage your tissues, accelerate aging and contribute to chronic disease.

KETOGENIC DIET

I talk a lot about a ketogenic diet in this book because of the miraculous health benefits it provides. This is a diet that helps shift your body's metabolic engine from burning carbohydrates to burning fats. Interestingly, the cells of your body have the metabolic flexibility to adapt from using glucose for fuel to using ketones, which are a byproduct of breaking down fats. We will talk about this more in the cancer section of this book, but cancer cells do not have this metabolic flexibility to use fat as energy. They require glucose to thrive, which makes a ketogenic diet so effective for treating and preventing cancer.

A ketogenic diet calls for minimizing carbohydrates and replacing them with healthy fats and moderate amounts of high-quality protein. A ketogenic diet requires that roughly 50 to 70 percent of your food intake come from healthy fats, such as avocado, coconut oil, grass-fed butter, organic pasture raised eggs, and raw nuts. This diet will also help optimize your weight and prevent virtually all chronic degenerative diseases. Because you are minimizing carbs and replacing them with healthy fats, your body will shift from burning carbs as your primary fuel to burning fat.

Dr. Peter Attia, a Stanford University trained physician specializing in metabolic science, applied the ketogenic diet to his lifestyle to see what would happen. He essentially used himself as a lab rat and received incredible results. Although he was an active and fit guy, he always had a tendency toward metabolic syndrome. Metabolic syndrome is a cluster of conditions – increased blood pressure, high blood sugar, excess body fat around the waist, and abnormal cholesterol or triglyceride levels – that occur together, increasing your risk of heart disease, stroke, and diabetes. He decided to experiment with the ketogenic diet and see if it could improve his overall health status.

He consumed 80 percent of his calories from fat for a period of 10 years and improved every measure of his health. MRI confirmed he didn't just lose an abundance of subcutaneous fat, but also the very harmful visceral fat around his organs. This demonstrates just how this diet can produce substantial changes in your body, even if you are believed to be physically fit. The following figure shows his lab levels before and after implementation of the ketogenic diet.

FIGURE 6.1: COMPARISON OF BLOOD MARKERS BEFORE AND AFTER IMPLEMENTATION OF A KETOGENIC DIET

	BEFORE	AFTER
Fasting blood sugar	100	75-95
Percentage body fat	25	10
Waist circumference in inches	40	31
Blood pressure	130/85	110/70
LDL	113	88
HDL	31	67
Triglycerides	152	22
Insulin sensitivity	Increased by more than 400 %	

Your heart and muscles operate very efficiently when they get the majority of their energy via ketones. Unlike your brain, your muscles actually store glucose in the form of glycogen for energy (See Chapter 3). Your brain, however, lacks this property, so it needs to find an alternate energy source.

When glucose is low, your brain tells your liver to produce ketones from fatty acids. Ketones are naturally produced in small amounts whenever you go for many hours without eating, such as after a full night's sleep. The liver will increase its production of ketones even further during fasting or when carbohydrate intake falls below 50 grams per day. When carbohydrates are limited, ketones can provide up to 70% of the brain's energy needs.

Even though most of the brain can use ketones, there are still some portions of the brain that require glucose to function properly. This can either come from the very small amounts of carbohydrates that is consumed during this diet, or a process your body can go through called gluconeogenesis, which means "making new glucose." Here, the liver creates glucose for the brain to use from amino acids, the building blocks of protein, and glycerol, a building block of fatty acids. This pathway ensures that the portions of the brain that need glucose will still get a steady supply, even when your carbohydrate intake is very low.

A ketone-like compound called beta-hydroxybutyrate (BHB) is made in abundance in the liver when in ketosis. This compound is able to efficiently fuel your brain. Interestingly, BHB also benefits the immune system. Researchers at the Yale School of Medicine observed that exposing human immune cells to BHB in amounts you would expect to find in the body following an intermittent fasting regimen for two days resulted in a reduced inflammatory response. This is a similar effect to abiding by the ketogenic diet for the same period of time. It also promoted recycling of damaged immune cells and the regeneration of new healthy immune cells. This just goes to show that short periods of fasting can support healthy immune function by promoting immune cell recycling and limiting the inflammatory response.

Ever wonder why you typically lose your appetite when you are sick? Interestingly, there is research supporting the idea that the lack of appetite you feel during the first few days of illness is your body's natural response and adaptation to fighting the infection. Three explanations exist for why this is true. First, from an evolutionary perspective, a lack of hunger eliminates the need to find food. This saves energy, decreases the amount of heat lost and allows the body to use its energy to focus solely on fighting the infection. Second, when we abstain from eating, we essentially deprive our body of the nutrients, such as iron and zinc, which help feed the infection of our body. This will prevent it from growing and spreading. Finally, the lack of appetite will encourage our body to recycle and remove infected cells through a process called apoptosis. This will be discussed in the next section.

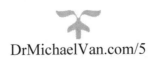

This beneficial effect from fasting when you are sick only has evidence of supporting your immune system during the acute phase of infection. This is why the lack of hunger when you are sick only lasts a few days and why most of us regain our normal appetite after the initial two days of our sickness.

Getting your body to burn ketones takes practice. The majority of the Western population has a diet very high in sugar and carbs, so they have completely lost their ability to burn ketones efficiently. With carbohydrates always present, your liver doesn't produce ketones because it has never needed to. The fat-burning engine has been completely shut off, even though many carry an enormous supply of it!

Think of this analogy. Imagine a large fuel truck carrying gas on a highway. As the fuel truck is running, it suddenly runs out of gas and stalls on the freeway. Even though the truck is carrying thousands of gallons of gas on board, this still can happen if the engine doesn't have the proper fuel. This happens to our body as well. Even though your body may have an abundant amount of fat stores, it doesn't have the capability to burn fat. It takes some re-training to burn fat for fuel. It is typically appropriate to start out by limiting your carbohydrates to 40 to 50 grams per day. This is easily attainable if we eliminate excess sugar and grains from our diet.

The difference between a ketogenic diet and a low-carb diet is that protein is often restricted in a ketogenic diet. The main goal of this diet is to increase blood levels of ketones, molecules that can partly replace carbohydrates as an energy source for the brain. Carbohydrate intake is limited to 50 grams or less with the ketogenic diet; in a low-carb diet, carb intake can vary form 25-150 grams per day.

KETOGENIC DIET AND ALZHEIMER'S DISEASE

The ketogenic diet provides many benefits for the brain. It appears to be very beneficial for people suffering from Alzheimer's disease, the most common form of dementia. It is classified as a progressive disease where the brain develops plaques and tangles that lead to memory loss. Many health experts consider Alzheimer's disease "type 3 diabetes," because the brain's cells become insulin resistant and are unable to use glucose properly, leading to inflammation.

There is a study on a group of 152 people with Alzheimer's disease that shows taking an MCT (Medium-Chain Triglyceride) supplement for 90 days increased ketone levels significantly and experienced a significant improvement in brain function. MCT is the type of medium chain fatty acid abundant in palm and coconut oil. Although the exact mechanism of why a ketogenic diet is effective is unclear, it appears to be due to the protection it gives brain cells by reducing reactive oxygen species (free radicals), which are the byproducts of metabolism and cause excess inflammation in the brain. In addition, the abundance of healthy fats also help reduce the level of harmful proteins that accumulate in the brains of people with Alzheimer's.

MULTI-SYSTEM REGENERATION

The journal *Cell Metabolism* described three major factors that happen when initiating intermittent fasting. First, this intermittent fasting regimen causes beneficial changes in risk factors of age-related diseases in humans, increasing lifespan. It rejuvenates the immune system and reduces cancer incidence. Finally, it actually promotes neurogenesis of the hippocampus and improves cognitive performance.

Intermittent fasting literally produced multi-system regeneration in mice and humans. This concept was discussed earlier in Chapter 5 when discussing brain function, but now we are going to look at this from the longevity perspective. Longevity and lifespan were significantly increased from this simple intervention due to many factors:

- Visceral belly fat, the harmful fat surrounding organs, was reduced

- The risk for cancer and inflammatory diseases declined

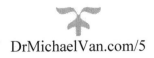

- Immune and brain function improved. In the mouse brain, neurons were regenerated, improving learning, memory, and concentration

- It also reduced the incidence of skin lesions and it ceased bone mineral density loss

- Intermittent fasting actually promoted healthy bone formation

To review the benefits we discussed earlier, see Figure 6.2 below.

FIGURE 6.2: MULTI-SYSTEM REGENERATION

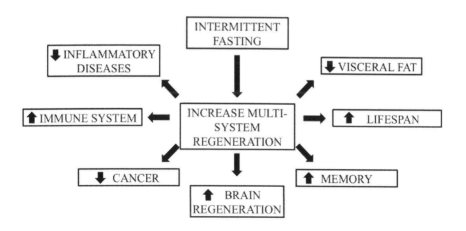

In part of this study discussing the pilot human trial, intermittent
fasting decreased risk factors and biomarkers for aging, diabetes,
cardiovascular disease, and cancer with no adverse side effects. The
authors actually concluded that this provides support for the use of
intermittent fasting not just to treat conditions like cancer, but to
promote health and extend lifespan, period.

FIGURE 6.3: RESULTS OF THE HUMAN TRIAL

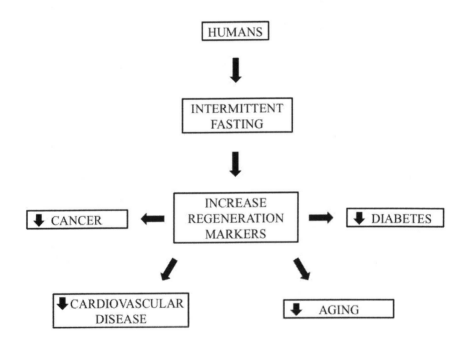

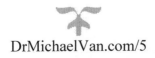

TOP 10 CAUSES OF DEATH

Here we go. I find it absolutely mind-blowing when I look at the top ten causes of death in the United States. Who would have thought that by doing an intervention like intermittent fasting, you could actually significantly reduce your risk of the top two causes of death in the world, which are heart disease (cardiovascular disease) and cancer? Not to mention the reduction of diabetes, which is currently the seventh leading cause of death. Looking at the research done on asthma patients and intermittent fasting, it wouldn't be a stretch to say that it significantly reduces the likelihood of developing chronic respiratory diseases as well, which is the third leading cause of death.

In our discussion on brain function, we know intermittent fasting dramatically reduces your risk of all neurodegenerative conditions, such as Alzheimer's, the sixth leading cause of death. We know from the abundance of research on intermittent fasting and its effect on inflammation, insulin sensitivity, blood pressure, and cholesterol, that it not only prevents heart disease, but also prevents stroke. Strokes are the fifth leading cause of death.

Therefore, by just incorporating a lifestyle change like intermittent fasting, you will reduce your risk of at least six of the top

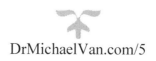

DrMichaelVan.com/5

ten leading causes of death in the United States. I can't explain how significant that is. What's frustrating is that doctors out there would rather give you a pill or worse, a surgery, to relieve your symptoms, to lower your expression of health, to increase the toxicity of the body, instead of recommending a proven intervention like intermittent fasting. Of course, like with many 'natural' interventions and lifestyle changes, they are simply not aware of this amazing eating pattern. It isn't part of the allopathic paradigm they practice in, where the goal of treatment options are only aimed at lowering symptoms. Intermittent fasting doesn't just prevent these diseases, it actually can be utilized as a treatment for each one of these conditions. In addition, it dramatically increases your expression of health and wellness, period.

STEM CELLS

What I find interesting in regards to longevity is exactly how intermittent fasting works to achieve this. The study out of the journal *Cell Stem Cell* helps explain it, intermittent fasting activates certain pathways in the body that help cells become stronger and more resistant to toxins. It was shown to completely reverse weakened immune systems and age-related disorders.

This study, along with a team of researchers from the University of Southern California, have found that intermittent fasting also significantly increases the regeneration of stem cells. It activates stem cells to promote self-renewal, making our immune systems much more efficient. Intermittent fasting literally enhances the ability of stem cells to divide and make more stem cells, allowing the body to effectively regenerate itself and stay healthy.

In an adult, stem cells are found in tissues and organs; they serve as the purpose of allowing the body to renew itself. These amazing cells are responsible for the maintenance and repair of tissues located where these stem cells are found. For example, we have blood-forming stem cells, called hematopoietic stem cells, located in our bone marrow. They are responsible for the constant maintenance and immune protection of every cell type of the body. These specialized blood cells allow for the constant renewal of blood, producing billions of new blood cells each day. Part of the explanation of why this regeneration of stem cells occurs is because the body becomes a lot more efficient when it switches to burning fat as fuel instead of glucose.

AUTOPHAGY

This next section can get a little confusing, but bear with me. Research has confirmed that intermittent calorie restriction helps extend lifespan and longevity by improving both insulin sensitivity and specific protective mechanisms in the nervous system.

Your brain and nervous system routinely go through a process of cellular cleansing, known as autophagy. Autophagy describes the process of the natural mechanism where neurons disassemble unnecessary or dysfunctional cellular components. It is a vital process where the body essentially begins to eat itself in an orderly pattern to remove damaged parts from your body. It allows the orderly degradation and recycling of cellular components, just like our body is constantly regenerating itself to stay healthy and fresh. In fact, many beauty products are put on the market to enhance autophagy, such as skin cells, in order to regenerate the cells and make it healthier and more protective.

What is neat is that intermittent fasting has actually been shown to dramatically up-regulate the process of autophagy, specifically in our brain and nerve cells. This was the first study of its kind to demonstrate that food restriction can lead to neuronal autophagy. Short term starvation (intermittent fasting) removes toxic molecules and damaged mitochondria from our brain cells. Mitochondria is known as the powerhouses of the cell. They are the working structures in the cell that keeps the cell full of energy. When this vital process of autophagy occurs in the mitochondria, it is called mitophagy. For simplicity, we are going to stick with the general term autophagy.

Enhanced autophagy from intermittent fasting improves longevity, as well as neuronal and brain function. The observed improvement of nervous system function is in part related to the up-regulation of autophagy. Although autophagy sounds like something you may want to avoid, it is actually the process that promotes health by cleaning house of all the impurities in the body. According to Colin Champ, M.D. and certified radiation oncologist at the University of Pittsburgh Medical Center:

> *"Think of it as our body's innate recycling program. Autophagy makes us more efficient machines to get rid of faulty parts, stop cancerous growths, and stop metabolic dysfunction like obesity and diabetes."*

Autophagy occurs at the cellular level where membranes break down. Your body recycles the healthy components, and it uses the rest

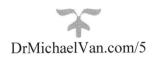

for energy to make new parts. Scientists engineered rats that were incapable of autophagy, the rats grew up with less energy, they were fatter, and they had impaired brain function.

In total, there are three distinct ways to elevate your body's ability to destroy worn out cells and regenerate new ones (the process of autophagy).:

1. Exercise - As mentioned before, it puts the body under stress by breaking down muscle and helping your body rebuild new tissue.

2. Intermittent fasting - It improves cognitive function, brain structure, and helps you learn more easily.

3. High fat diet - This diet should consist mainly of high quality healthy fats, with moderate levels of high quality protein and minimal amounts of non-fiber carbohydrates. Quality fats include avocado, grass-fed meats, grass-fed butter from a local farmer (Kerry Gold if purchased from a grocery store), organic pastured egg yolks, coconut oil, and raw nuts and seeds. The idea here is to limit carbohydrate intake to levels where your body has no other choice but to burn fat as fuel.

FIGURE 6.4: KETOGENIC DIET BREAKDOWN

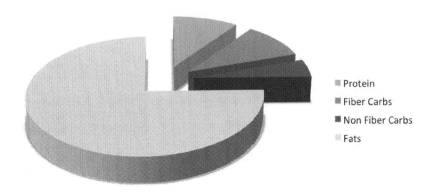

What this diet on the above pie chart consists of is 10% protein, 10% fiber carbohydrates, 5% non-fiber carbohydrates, and 75% healthy fats. This type of diet helps your body fight off cancer, lower your risk of diabetes, fight off some brain disorders, and reduce seizures in children.

Monitoring protein intake here is just as important as cutting down non-vegetable carbohydrates. If you consume more protein than

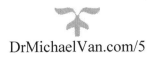

DrMichaelVan.com/5

your body needs, then you will actually prevent the activation of stem cells and the regeneration of your immune system. Too much protein in your body increases the mTOR, PKA, and IGF pathways in the body that will block the above benefits to stem cells and autophagy.

Intermittent fasting reduces the amount of IGF-1 (Insulin-like growth factor-1), a hormone similar to insulin. Intermittent fasting and the diet outlined above lead to lower blood levels of the hormones insulin and IGF-1. This results in an increase of stem cell self-renewal and reverses immunosuppression. Together, this actually increases cell regeneration and causes cancer cells to get less signals to grow and divide.

FIGURE 6.5: INTERMITTENT FASTING AND LONGEVITY

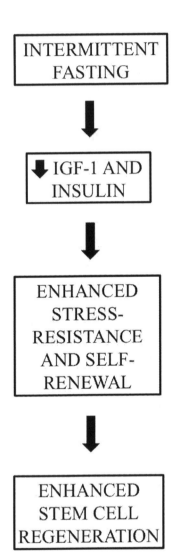

What is also interesting is that a lack of autophagy results in neurodegenerative diseases, or diseases caused by a breakdown of your brain and nerve cells. Examples of neurodegenerative diseases are Alzheimer's disease, Huntington disease, and Parkinson's disease. This is encouraging because researches are constantly trying to develop drugs that can enhance neuron autophagy, thereby protecting you against disease. It is just so difficult to make a drug with this capability because it must meet three criteria:

1. These drugs need to be able to cross the blood-brain barrier to reach the brain and nervous system in the first place.

2. The drugs need to be able to enhance and up-regulate neuronal autophagy.

3. The drugs need to be harmless to the recipient (*like that will ever happen.* Drugs have a long list of side effects for a reason).

Intermittent fasting represents an attractive alternative to drug therapy without any harmful symptoms. It provides a natural process that our body is designed for to promote healthy longevity, anti-aging, and brain protective properties that can't be simulated in a lab.

The bottom line is that intermittent fasting has very promising evidence that shows its anti-aging and longevity properties. Depending on the study, intermittent fasting has been shown to increase lifespan in rats by as much as 36-83% longer. It improves your immune system and mitochondrial function, reduces your inflammatory process and the amount of free radicals in your body, and slows down the aging process significantly, especially if eating your macronutrients in the ratios in the pie chart above in figure 6.4. Going without food now and then will not kill you. In fact, it is one of the keys to living a longer and healthier life.

MICROBIOME CHANGES

We have already illustrated the fact that intermittent fasting promotes an increase in your lifespan. Driving the point home even further, it has also been shown to elicit major changes in your gut bacteria or microflora in ways that promote longevity.

The microflora, located in the intestines and other parts of your digestive system, are made up of approximately 100 trillion cells. In fact, your gut bacteria actually outnumber the other cells of the body at a ratio of nearly 10:1. It is true that most disease processes originate in your digestive system, and include diseases that impact your brain, your heart, your weight, and your immune system. Not surprisingly, there is also specific microorganisms in your gut that directly affect the aging process, and this is exactly what brought this new research to light on the relationship between fasting and longevity.

Remember, your gut bacteria is not static. The microbes in your gut are always changing in response to your environment. Simply put, when you fill your lifestyle with healthy choices, you alter your gut to promote longevity and health. When you fill your lifestyle with unhealthy choices, you alter your gut bacteria to promote the beginning of disease and sickness. By far, one of the largest influences on the quality of your microflora is your diet and your dieting patterns.

Continuous calorie restriction is not a compelling and popular method for most people due to the lack of willingness to deprive yourself of calories to the level required to get these health benefits. Therefore, intermittent fasting is a much more acceptable option. Recent research suggests that intermittent calorie restriction, such as simply restricting your daily eating window, may offer many of these same benefits as continuous fasting. These benefits include increasing lifespan and preventing chronic disease.

It is not surprising then that a study titled, "Effects of Intermittent Feeding Upon Growth and Life Span in Rats," showed a significant increase in lifespan in rats who were put on an intermittent fasting regimen. The lifespan of rats in the intermittent fasting group represented an 83% increase over the group of rats maintained on an ad libitum diet (eating whenever they wanted). By simply changing the pattern of eating, life span can potentially increase by 83%! How cool (and simple) is that?

By radically improving your beneficial gut bacteria, you will be dramatically improving your immune function due to the fact that your

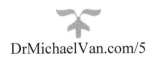

microflora makes up 80% of your immune system. Not only does this happen when you optimize your bacteria, but you will sleep better, have more energy, have greater mental clarity, and concentrate better.

It has even been shown in the recent journals *Nature* and *Science* that optimizing your gut bacteria down regulates the development of lymphoma, a cancer of the white blood cells. In addition, a healthy gut has also been shown to decrease a specific inflammatory response that fuels the development and growth of some cancers. This inflammation caused by poor gut bacteria allows pathogens, such as E.coli, to invade your gut and cause cellular damage. That means that replenishing your good bacteria is important for the prevention of virtually all disease, from colds to cancer. To summarize, essentially every aspect of your life and health will improve when you begin the process of optimizing your gut microflora.

As you know, intermittent fasting is not the only intervention that can optimize your microflora for better health. Other of my recommendations include adding:

- Fermented Foods
  - This is by far the best route to attain optimal digestive health. Healthy choices include fermented vegetables, such as kimchi and sauerkraut, as well as grass-fed organic milk, such as kefir. One tablespoon of this will actually contain more healthy probiotics than a full bottle of most high-quality probiotic supplements, making it cost effective as well. On average, most probiotic supplements contain no more than 10 billion colony-forming units, where one serving of fermented vegetables can contain 10 trillion colony-forming units of bacteria. Fermented foods also give you more of a variety of beneficial microbes.

- Probiotic Supplement
  - I am personally not a fan of many supplements as I believe most nutrients need to come from food; however, a probiotic supplement is an exception. They should be

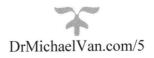

taken if you do not consume fermented foods on a daily basis.

It is also just as important to know exactly what to avoid to achieve optimal gut bacteria. This includes avoiding:

- Antibiotics
  - There are exceptions to every rule, but generally you want to avoid these unless absolutely necessary. If you do choose to use them, it is important to make sure you take it with fermented foods and/or a probiotic supplement to help replenish your gut.

- Conventionally Raised Meats
  - This includes all animal products from concentrated animal feeding operations (CAFO). It is routine to feed low-dose antibiotics to these animals that aid in the destruction of your gut. Coupled with genetically engineered grains that the animals consume, this makes CAFO animals very dangerous.

- Processed Foods
  - Processed foods such as excessive amounts of grains and sugars feed your pathogenic bacteria.

- Agricultural Chemicals
  - This includes glyphosate, a neurotoxin, found in RoundUp. Unless the food is 100% organic, it is likely it contains GMO's that are heavily contaminated with pesticides.

- Chlorinated And / Or Fluoridated Water
  - Chlorine / fluoride kills not only the pathogenic bacteria in water but it also kills the beneficial bacteria in your gut.

- Antibacterial Soaps
  - These soaps you wash your bodies and hands with kill off both your bad and good bacteria, and overtime can contribute to antibiotic resistance. This also includes antibacterial hand sanitizers. Even though they are not consumed, they still destroy the good bacteria on the skin and get absorbed into the bloodstream.

Aside from the beneficial impact on your gut microflora, many of the anti-aging and longevity benefits stem from the massive increases you get from enhanced human growth hormone (HGH) production. As stated before, intermittent fasting has been linked to a 1,300% increase in human growth hormone secretion in women, and an astounding 2,000% increase in men! This statistic is so mind-blowing that I had to state it again. HGH, commonly known as your fitness hormone, plays a huge role in maintaining health, fitness, and longevity. All of these properties are absolutely essential for anti-aging and longevity, keeping your body running at optimum performance until the latter years of your life!

CHAPTER 7:

THE mTOR PATHWAY

The proper regulation of the mTOR (mammalian target of rapamycin) protein is another key way to extend lifespan. The mTOR gene plays a role in cellular metabolism and energy balance and holds the key to muscle building and rejuvenation. Dysregulation in our mTOR pathway leads to accelerated aging, muscle wasting, and early mortality.

In the 2013 issue of the journal *Cell Reports*, scientists discovered that the mTOR gene is a significant regulator of the aging process. When mice were given a drug called rapamycin, an immunosuppressant used to treat cancer patients that down-regulates this mTOR gene, they lived 20% longer than the mice in the control group not given this gene. In human terms, this equates to nearly 15 years of additional life! The other beneficial effects of down-regulating this mTOR gene included improved memory, cognition, and a much lower cancer risk.

With that being said, there were other effects this drug produced that were not so good. The fact of the matter is, all drugs come with harmful side effects. The mTOR-suppressed mice from the rapamycin medication exhibited side effects that included softer bones, more infections, muscle wasting, and more cataracts than normal mice. This brought a new challenge into the spotlight: to figure out how to *naturally* optimize this mTOR pathway in order to reap the benefits of increased lifespan without any of the negative side effects like muscle wasting. Obviously, an increase in lifespan combined with limited muscle mass would be counterintuitive, because muscle mass is essential for having a high quality of life. Therefore, the search for how to maximize both longevity and human performance at the same time needed to be conducted.

What researchers discovered in response to this challenge is that fasting, diet, and exercise can significantly enhance our mTOR pathways. They discovered that mTOR is closely related to our insulin pathway. When insulin is released, it up-regulates our mTOR pathway.

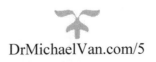

Put another way, if we give our body just the right amount of insulin it needs to thrive, our mTOR pathways will be properly activated. Excessive insulin release from chronically poor diets and a lack of exercise, on the other hand, wreaks havoc to our mTOR pathways, and thus to our health and lifespan.

Here is an example. When it comes to insulin signaling, we have many similarities with animals. Adding a tiny amount of glucose to a worm's normal diet caused its lifespan to shorten by 20 percent. This was all due to the resulting increase in glucose above normal levels, leading to higher levels of insulin above normal conditions. The increased amounts of insulin, above normal levels, decreased insulin sensitivity and down-regulated the worms' mTOR activity. Humans follow the same pattern. This is why I have been saying the same thing for years: consuming excess sugar and grains throughout your life is the equivalent of slamming your foot on the accelerator for aging.

Since mTOR is part of the insulin pathway, we need to look at the action of insulin to fully understand the function of the mTOR protein. You don't always want insulin at very low levels. Instead, you want it to be very responsive. You want it to be very sensitive. We need insulin to function correctly in order to be healthy. It is essential for life. After all, it is one of our anabolic hormones that builds the body up and brings energy in the form of glucose into our cells.

It is essential that insulin stays at optimal levels based on the body's demand. In times of feeding, insulin levels rise to feed our cells. It then lowers in the periods in between feeding to keep insulin sensitivity at its peak. Insulin resistance, from chronically elevated insulin levels, is detrimental to your health and leads to chronic disease. This is almost always due to a chronically poor diet consisting of processed carbohydrates in combination with a lack of exercise. When you lose your normal insulin sensitivity, you also lose your ability to effectively utilize the mTOR pathway and get the desired results of increased lifespan and lean muscle mass.

The good news is intermittent fasting and exercise enhance our mTOR pathway by naturally inhibiting it temporarily. This period of inhibition is vital for our health in the same way it is vital for our insulin to be inhibited when we are not eating. mTOR is then activated and at its peak responsiveness right after exercise and fasting in order to properly stimulate protein synthesis in your muscles. The lack of food and intense bouts of exercise down-regulate this pathway temporarily to give us the increased lifespan benefits. The periods after fasting and

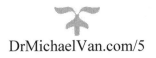

exercise up-regulate the action of this pathway to give us the proper muscle building benefits we need for optimal human performance.

FIGURE 7.1: REGULATORS OF mTOR ACTIVITY

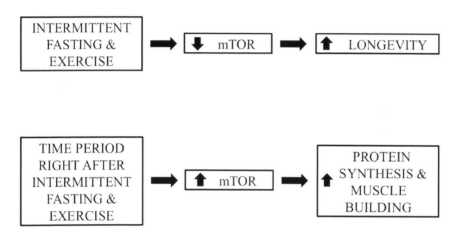

This is exactly what we want as humans. We want this pathway to be down-regulated throughout our fasting period so it can produce a major spike right after our fasting period or workout. This major spike that occurs will allow our body to reap all the benefits of increased protein synthesis and muscle building. The time period we are fasting in will cause this pathway to be down-regulated, giving us the longer lifespan we all yearn to have. In this way, we have successfully figured out the challenge presented above: to figure out how to *naturally*

optimize this mTOR pathway in order to increase both lifespan and healthy muscle mass. This "balance," if you will, of a properly functioning mTOR pathway is crucial for health and longevity.

THE mTOR PATHWAY AND MUSCLE BUILDING

As mentioned before, the mTOR pathway is crucial for regulating muscle protein synthesis and breakdown. I believe that muscle retention is the most critical element of human fitness. Healthy amounts of skeletal muscle play an important biological role in keeping you strong, functional and healthy. It not only helps you produce physical movement, but it also helps regulate glucose and lipid metabolism and increases your insulin sensitivity. It protects you against obesity, diabetes, cardiovascular disease and any other chronic disease.

Muscle wasting, on the other hand, is due to a lack of adequate exercise, disease or aging. It leads to the loss of physical capacity, loss of physical shape, and an increased risk of chronic disease. Therefore, triggering this innate muscle building mechanism is extremely important.

The absolute key muscle building mechanism in all mammals is this complex pathway called the mTOR. When mTOR is activated, it signals your muscle to increase protein synthesis. When mTOR is inhibited, your muscle protein synthesis shuts down and protein breakdown increases. The ratio here of protein synthesis/protein breakdown is what is important. It will determine whether you build or waste muscle.

mTOR ACTIVATORS

There are three main triggers of the mTOR pathway. These include fasting, exercise and proper intake of branched-chain amino acids (BCAA's). Fasting reduces your body's insulin activity, giving your body time to heal cell membranes and improve insulin receptor sensitivity. It also allows the body to detoxify itself from wastes, old proteins, and other weakened and damaged cellular compounds. Fasting gives your body the chance to rest and rejuvenate itself. It increases insulin sensitivity so we can promote maximized healing, growth, and repair of our muscles and tissues.

The mTOR pathway responds to exercise in a similar fashion. During exercise, your mTOR pathway is completely inhibited. The period after exercise, however, it gets reactivated and is further enhanced by amino acids and insulin. Since mTOR is crucial for muscle growth, consuming proper nutrition immediately after exercise will help the mTOR pathway boost muscle protein synthesis to levels greater than protein breakdown. This will result in a net gain of healthy muscle mass.

Therefore, mTOR is inhibited while your body is in a fasted state and during exercise, but gets reactivated upon feeding and the period

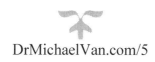

DrMichaelVan.com/5

right after your workout. You basically shift from a catabolic or breakdown state to an anabolic or build-up state. Both exercise and fasting cause muscle protein breakdown initially, but then both will radically stimulate protein synthesis at the times right after intense exercise and feeding.

THE CASE FOR HIGH-INTENSITY INTERVAL TRAINING

Exercise also optimizes mTOR activity, but not all types of exercise are equal. The type of exercise or mechano-overload that is proven to enhance mTOR is a training technique called high-intensity interval training (HIIT). This link http://bit.ly/2adTYGE will take you to my detailed video on this topic. This very intense type of workout regimen turns your mTOR pathways into turbo mode, increasing protein synthesis in your muscle fibers. HIIT performed directly after fasting creates a natural anabolic state in your body. In addition, it dramatically improves insulin signaling within muscle cells, further increasing the action of mTOR. HIIT also happens to be the form of exercise that boosts human growth hormone levels the most, which gives your body powerful anti-aging effects. Applying this training method will lead to an increase in muscle size and longevity.

Low to moderate intensity exercise such as long-distance aerobics cannot achieve this. Just look at the body type and muscle mass difference between a world-class sprinter versus a long distance marathon runner. Moderate exercise simply lacks the proper intensity that is needed to stimulate mTOR and hence make this huge muscle building impact.

On a side note, what is even worse is that chronic prolonged aerobics, like long-distance running, can actually lead to a loss of muscle size and strength. The key word here is 'chronic.' Researchers in the field of muscle biology and aging have actually found evidence of the connection between prolonged aerobic activity and an increase in oxidative damage in your muscles. Prolonged aerobics causes a massive accumulation of free radicals in your muscles, which can eventually lead to oxidative damage. Of course, if you have a balanced training regimen that calls for resistance training three times a week and running four miles two to three times a week, that is perfectly ok.

What makes short bouts of intense exercise superior in terms of oxidative damage is that your body is able to counteract the oxidative stress without depleting the antioxidant stores in your body. Essentially, the resting periods between each major bout of intense exercise gives your muscles time to recuperate. Again, it also has been shown to yield the perfect scenario to trigger the mTOR pathway and increase muscle mass. High intensity interval training should be short in duration in the range of 5-30 minutes to keep oxidative stress from causing too much damage. Overtraining or exercising at this high intensity for longer durations can lead to excessive oxidative damage and stress, causing the body to secrete cortisol. Cortisol, a stress hormone, is catabolic in

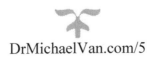

nature, so it leads to the body breaking down instead of the desired anabolic effect of building up.

The other reason why intense exercise is superior is that it works directly on your fast twitch muscle fibers, also known as your type IIA and type IIB fibers. These fast twitch muscle fibers enable you to perform powerful, strong, and fast movements, and give you the capacity to generate lots of force. These are also the fibers that are most prone to damage and wasting, especially as you age. They enable you to climb stairs, lift heavy grocery bags, move furniture, etc. Your fast twitch fibers make up roughly 50% or more of your muscles diameter, and are only maintained and kept intact by intense exercise.

In contrast, your slow twitch muscle fibers, your type I fibers, are the muscles most people work from prolonged aerobics and aren't as prone to damage, wasting, and degradation as you age. These are the muscle fibers worked when you walk at a steady state, or even do excessive long distance aerobic activity. These activities are not bad as long as you are also doing specific high intensity exercises to stimulate your type II fibers. When you don't use your fast twitch muscle fibers and give them the proper stimulation they need, they begin to atrophy or shrink in size. You know what they say: if you don't use it, you lose it.

THE WINDOW OF OPPORTUNITY

The third and final trigger of your mTOR pathway is proper nutritional triggers, especially right after your bout of exercise is completed. That is why roughly 30 minutes after an intense workout is known as the "window of opportunity." This time period serves as your big chance to maximize your mTOR activity in order to get the most out of your fasting and exercise periods.

The nutritional triggers that stimulate mTOR and muscle growth are branched chain amino acids (BCAA's). These amino acids are the major players in muscle building. What this means is that consuming high-quality protein that contains the proper amounts of BCAA's within 30 minutes or so after a workout will increase the rate of muscle protein synthesis after exercise and simultaneously lower the rate of muscle protein breakdown.

Let's break this concept down. Complete dietary protein provides the nine essential amino acids your body needs for muscle growth. The most important amino acids out of this group that stimulate your mTOR are your three BCAA's, which include leucine, isoleucine, and valine. The most important amino acid out of the three BCAA's is leucine. Unlike other amino acids that serve as building blocks to

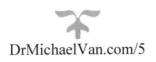

protein, branched chain amino acids (especially leucine) also signal your muscles to increase protein synthesis.

The protein I recommend right after a workout is a high quality grass-fed whey protein concentrate powder. This type of protein contains the highest concentration of BCAA's, especially leucine. It is estimated we need around 1-3 grams a day of total leucine to maintain our body protein, and around 8-16 grams a day of leucine to optimize our muscle building anabolic pathway and promote muscle building. Therefore, to establish the perfect anabolic or muscle building environment for your muscles, we need to increase leucine and BCAA consumption beyond maintenance requirements. Food based supplementation is always superior for proper absorption without side effects.

In order to get the minimum eight grams of leucine to properly stimulate mTOR, you would need to consume one of the following amounts of food:

- A pound and a half of chicken
- Three pounds of pork
- Over a pound of almonds
- 16 eggs

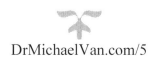

- Half a pound of raw cheddar cheese

If this amount of food seems difficult, you are not alone. There is no way I'm going to eat three pounds of pork right after working out to satisfy my leucine requirement! I would explode! The good news is that you can also get this amount of leucine from only three ounces of high-quality whey protein. That is why whey protein supplementation is the best option to get the recommended amounts of BCAA's you need to build muscle without consuming an enormous amount of food that can actually hinder your health.

These special amino acids have shown the ability to stimulate muscle protein synthesis even during times of food restriction or fasting. This is why I also recommend consuming a high quality BCAA supplement before a bout of exercise, especially if you are exercising in a fasted state. Exercising in a fasted state promotes massive growth hormone production as well as optimal fat burning and muscle building.

Remember, in order to optimize your mTOR pathway for an increase in healthy muscle mass, you must have optimal insulin sensitivity and glucose balance, which I like to call the glycemic factor. The mTOR pathway is very responsive to hormonal stimulation, particularly to an optimal balance of glucose, insulin, and IGF-1

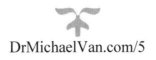

(insulin-like growth factor-1). IGF-1 is stimulated by growth hormone and intense exercise, but it needs just the right amount of insulin to finalize its role. All of this comes into play during the recovery period right after a bout of intense exercise.

The perfect time to feed the body, in order to promote muscle gain, is right after exercise. Insulin from the post-workout meal is able to kick in while IGF-1 and human growth hormone are already at their peak from the high intensity exercise. All these factors work together to massively stimulate healthy mTOR activity. Impaired glucose and insulin activity, such as insulin resistance, inactivates your mTOR and will inhibit your muscle building capability. Not only that, insulin resistance is just bad for your health, period, and leads to every chronic disease on the planet. That is why all three activators of your mTOR (fasting, high intensity exercise, BCAA's) work together to promote insulin sensitivity in order for our body's to exhibit peak performance.

THE DANGER OF TOO MANY CARBS

To optimize insulin and glucose when it comes to triggering mTOR and muscle mass, the topic again goes back to BCAA's from a high quality whey protein source. Consuming this within 30 minutes after a workout is crucial because they actually contribute carbon molecules to an energy cycle called the alanine glucose cycle (for the science people out there, this is part of the Kreb's Cycle). BCAA's actually donate a carbon to this pathway, and in the process synthesize glucose to supply your muscles. This pathway is special because it makes just enough glucose to meet the needs of your muscle tissues, and no more. This way you won't get a huge spike of glucose or insulin that occurs when we get our fuel after a workout from too many carbohydrates. Too many carbohydrates hinder insulin sensitivity and as a result will hinder your mTOR.

This physiological process mainly occurs in the liver, giving your body the perfect amount of glucose to feed your muscles during intermittent fasting and exercise. Your liver makes the perfect amount of glucose that your muscles require. This mechanism of fueling your muscles with amino acids and protein is so efficient that your blood sugar will never spike. It is possible that we even evolved to acquire this perfect protein fueling mechanism during Paleolithic times. These were

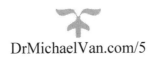

the times when humans were performing extreme physical activity (mimicked by high intensity training) while maintaining a diet/lifestyle that consisted of healthy fats, protein, and devoid of grains and sugar (the diet our body's are made for).

On the other hand, high carbohydrate meals shut down this primal fueling mechanism. This causes your body to use the less effective fuel in the form of carbohydrates. Although endurance athletes such as long distance runners can benefit from complex carbohydrate loading, there is too much evidence on the contrary showing how our human body was not evolved to work well on a diet high in carbohydrates.

Recent studies show that adding simple carbohydrates to your protein supplements actually negate the muscle building effects of the whey protein. That is a huge problem today in the fitness world. People buy into the concept of 'muscle fueling' with high glycemic carbohydrate fuel and have completely shifted away from the low glycemic fat and protein fuel we were evolved to consume. Now we are paying the consequences with growing rates of diabetes, metabolic syndrome, and obesity.

THE SCIENTIFIC APPROACH TO
INTERMITTENT FASTING

In a recent study in the *Journal of Physiology*, it indicated that performing exercise in a fasted state with a low glycemic post workout meal (or shake) promotes fat loss as well as muscle gain. Your glycemic index, or glycemic load, is a measure of how your blood glucose levels increase after consuming foods. Low glycemic foods are types of foods that do not cause your blood sugar to spike, such as healthy fats, protein and low glycemic fruits like berries. This study also showed that eating the same meal before exercise instead of after actually caused fat gain and less protein synthesis in your muscle, showing that this idea of a pre-workout meal is not necessarily based on science. On the contrary, those who were intermittent fasting before their workout increased their insulin sensitivity and maximized their mTOR pathway.

Therefore, to get healthy and put on lean muscle mass, you need to maximize your mTOR pathway. This means intermittent fasting and eating low glycemic foods we were originally programmed for. Fasting stimulates a huge spike in muscle protein synthesis once feeding is resumed. Increasing your intake of leucine rich foods and other branched chain amino acids from high quality whey protein and organic pasture-raised eggs complements intermittent fasting for developing and maintaining healthy muscle mass.

Feed your muscles with quality whey protein concentrate after exercise derived from grass fed cows that is ideally cold processed. The brand of whey protein that I personally have been consuming is Naked Whey, which is a grass fed whey protein powder from California Farms. Whey protein's anabolic impact after exercise is unmatched. As a general rule, keep your protein total to around 20 grams, because this is around the threshold level needed for maximum utilization and bioavailability without your body wasting nitrogen. It is ok to mix your protein with low glycemic fruit, like berries. One trick to help maximize leucine's effect on the anabolic process is adding coconut oil to your whey protein. These medium chain fatty acids in coconut oil help give you instant energy without spiking insulin and can actually help you shift leucine's pathway from fueling into muscle building.

CHAPTER 8:

IMPROVED INSULIN SENSITIVITY

Insulin is a hormone produced by the beta cells of your pancreas. It is secreted in small amounts throughout the day and in larger amounts after a meal is consumed. When we eat a meal that contains carbohydrates, your blood sugar begins to increase. Since blood sugar cannot go into your cells directly, it needs insulin. Your pancreas senses the rise in blood sugar, and releases insulin as a result. Insulin then binds to cells, which signals them to absorb the sugar from the bloodstream. Insulin is often referred to as the key that unlocks the cell to allow sugar to enter and be used for energy.

If you have more sugar than your body needs, insulin helps store it in your liver or muscle in the form of glycogen. This way, when your blood sugar levels become low, you will have extra stores in your liver that can be released back into the bloodstream. (Stored glycogen in your muscle is unable to get released in the bloodstream like your liver because it lacks a specific enzyme). The role of insulin is to regulate blood sugar levels and keep them into the normal range. Every time blood sugar rises, your pancreas will secrete more insulin.

INSULIN AND FAT STORAGE

The problem arises when insulin becomes chronically elevated in the body. Insulin happens to be the main fat storage hormone in the body. It tells fat cells to store fat, and it prevents stored fat from being broken down for energy. Think about it this way. Insulin can only be present in the blood if we have elevated blood sugar. We can only have elevated blood sugar if we recently consumed a meal. Therefore, if we are in an energetic surplus from recently consuming a meal, insulin gets released to store this available energy. The last thing the body will want to do in this situation is breakdown its energy stores in the form of fat for energy, because we already have energy.

What happens when a department store gets a shipment of product in? Do they release the stored inventory they already have? No. They are in storage or surplus mode. The workers take the shipment and store it within the store where there is room. The only time they can actually get rid of and use the stored materials and inventory they have is if they cut down the number of shipments of product and use what they already have.

It is the same with the body. When we have a shipment of glucose from a recently consumed meal, our body is turned into storage

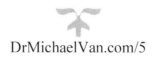

mode and insulin gets released to store all the energy we recently consumed. The only time you can actually start burning your stored energy located in your fat stores is if we stop eating and allow our body to utilize the energy it already has.

When people are obese or are chronically eating a diet filled with processed foods and fast burning carbohydrates, insulin is constantly being released by the pancreas. Eventually, our cells stop responding to the increase in insulin. In other words, the cells become resistant or numb to the increased insulin. When this occurs, the pancreas still does its job (for the time being) by detecting more and more increases in blood sugar. In turn, the pancreas then releases more and more insulin into the blood stream to bring the blood sugar levels down. The problem is that the insulin receptors on cells don't respond and are not sensitive to the rise in insulin anymore. They become insulin resistant.

The end result is chronically high amounts of insulin in the blood, called hyperinsulinemia, and chronically elevated blood sugar, called hyperglycemia. Do you think this person is able to burn its fat stores? Not a chance! They are in constant energy surplus mode. The chronic elevated insulin levels in the body will not allow the breakdown of fat stores, resulting in the person getting more and more obese.

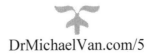

FIGURE 8.1: INSULIN RESISTANCE

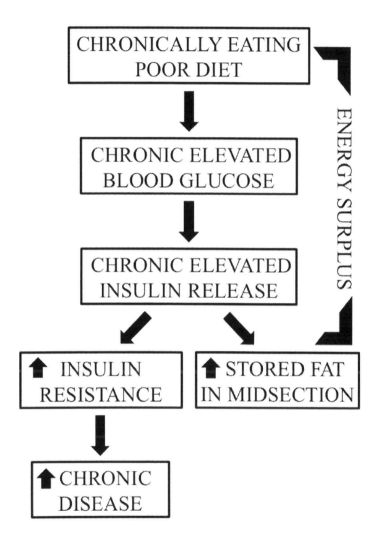

Chronic elevated insulin levels isn't the only thing that happens when we are in a chronic stressful environment of unhealthy eating and a lack of exercise. This also leads to a chronic release of stress hormones, putting your body in a chronic stress response. These hormones increase heart rate, cardiac output, and blood pressure. They down regulate all the processes in the body that have to do with growth and repair and up regulate all the processes that have to do with body breakdown. Stress hormones down-regulate your immune system and increase cholesterol in your blood because cholesterol is the precursors to hormone production. They cause the hippocampus of your brain to shrink and decrease your ability to sleep. You will get tension headaches, have decreased sex drive, get low levels of growth hormone, and continue to crave sugar and unhealthy fats.

Stress hormones also further down regulate insulin receptors, not allowing the receptors to take blood sugar out of your bloodstream and into your cells. When this becomes chronic, it leads to type II diabetes, heart disease, obesity, cancer, and many other chronic conditions. The increase in glucose from a poor diet high in processed carbohydrates leads to further increases in insulin.   It decreases magnesium levels of the body, which is required for muscle relaxation, so blood vessels continue to constrict and get smaller, further increasing your blood pressure and putting stress on your cardiovascular system.

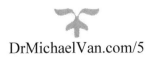

I like to think of insulin resistance as an annoying sound like a dog barking. At first, the sound is very annoying and you become very responsive at trying to remove yourself from that noise however possible. If the dog persists to bark and you can't do anything about it, you slowly start to become desensitized to the stimulus and stop trying to respond. You start to become numb to the sound, just like your cells start to become numb to the ever-increasing amounts of insulin.

Roughly 40% of the U.S. population is insulin resistant. In the United States, an estimated 70 million individuals are affected by insulin resistance. What is even more alarming is about a third or our children and teenagers are beginning to develop beginning stages of insulin resistance. Insulin sensitivity is the complete opposite of insulin resistance. If you are insulin resistant, then you have low insulin sensitivity. If you are insulin sensitive, you have low insulin resistance

A chronically poor diet leads to increased visceral fat, which is the dangerous belly fat that surrounds the organs of the body. This type of fat actually release fatty acids into the blood as well as inflammatory hormones that further drive insulin resistance. It becomes a very destructive never-ending cycle unless drastic lifestyle changes are implemented.

According to a study out of the *Journal of Laboratory and Clinical Medicine*, people lost 4-7% of their waist circumference from intermittent fasting. This indicates that they lost significant amounts of the harmful belly fat that builds up around the organs and causes disease.

Normal weight individuals can have insulin resistance; however, it is just much more common among those who are overweight. Excessive amounts of refined carbohydrates and sugars in your diet are among many other causes of insulin resistance. Additional notable causes are increased inflammation and oxidative stress in the body, physical inactivity and a disruption of the gut microflora.

Risk factors for insulin resistance are those who are overweight or obese, and especially those who have large amounts of fat in the midsection. Having low levels of HDL (high-density lipoprotein) and high blood triglycerides are two other markers strongly associated with insulin resistance.

INTERMITTENT FASTING AND INSULIN RESISTANCE

Apart from exercise, intermittent fasting is the most powerful natural insulin sensitizer known. Intermittent fasting also helps reverse the inflammation and the dysfunctional gut that contributes to insulin resistance as well.

In the study out of the *International Journal of Obesity*, Mattson and his colleagues found that intermittent fasting was effective at reducing inflammation, improving metabolic disease markers and reducing insulin resistance. These metabolic disease markers include reducing free fatty acids in the bloodstream, as well as increasing HDL and decreasing LDL.

The *American Journal of Clinical Nutrition, Journal of Applied Physiology, and The Journal of Nutritional Biochemistry* also showed a significant reduction in insulin resistance by intermittent fasting. By ceasing the development of insulin resistance through intermittent fasting, a proper diet and exercise, it will then prevent every other chronic disease out there, especially metabolic syndrome, type II diabetes and heart disease. In fact, people who are insulin resistant have a 93% greater risk for developing heart disease, the leading cause of

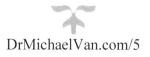

death in the world. The other diseases linked to insulin resistance
includes liver disease, polycystic ovarian syndrome, Alzheimer's
disease, and cancer.

Intermittent fasting gives our body a break from eating
throughout the day, turning our bodies from an energy surplus machine
into an energy deficit machine. When we take a break from constantly
feeding our body, our blood sugar begins to normalize. When we don't
have an increase in blood sugar, we will not release insulin. Since
insulin prevents fat stores from being burned, we will finally give our
body a chance to actually burn stored fat around the midsection and start
to build up our insulin sensitivity again. When we build up our insulin
sensitivity, we will begin to prevent every single chronic disease out
there, reducing our chances of heart disease by 93%!

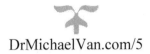

FIGURE 8.2: INTERMITTENT FASTING AND INSULIN

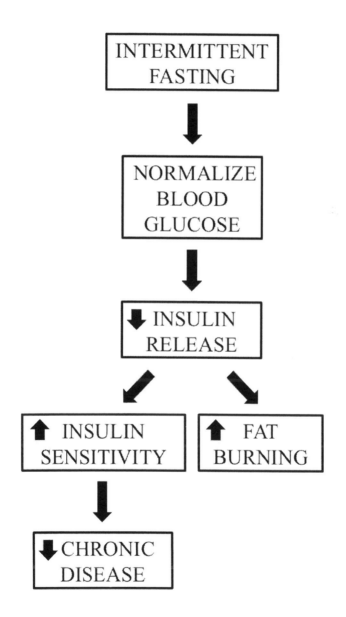

Remember what I said about human growth hormone in earlier chapters? Human growth hormone and insulin are indirectly related, so we as humans simply cannot release growth hormone when our insulin is chronically elevated. Intermittent fasting combats this problem by lowering insulin levels in the blood and using up our excessive harmful fat stores as energy. When you incorporate intermittent fasting, human growth hormone levels go up and insulin levels go down. You also change the expression of genes and initiate important cellular repair processes.

Insulin resistance can be completely reversed with simple lifestyle measures. Preventing insulin resistance with healthy lifestyle measures can be one of the most powerful lifestyle changes you make to live a longer, healthier and happier life.

CHAPTER 9:

INCREASED LEPTIN SENSITIVITY

Leptin is a hormone made by your fat cells that is responsible for reducing hunger. It is also known as your "satiety hormone" or the "master hormone of body fat regulation." When you eat a meal, leptin gets released by your fat cells and travels to the hypothalamus, a structure in the brain. It basically signals to your brain that your body is full and needs no more food. It is an important hormone that aids in appetite control. See the figure below for a brief summary of normal leptin function.

FIGURE 9.1: NORMAL LEPTIN FUNCTION

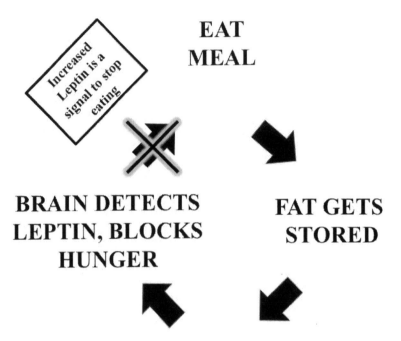

If it weren't for leptin, our bodies would constantly crave more and more food. Low leptin levels lead to an increase in hunger and a decrease in metabolic rate. High leptin leads to a decrease in hunger and an increase in metabolic rate. This is due to the intimate relationship between leptin and your thyroid hormones, which regulate metabolism, growth and development. When we eat a meal under normal conditions, leptin rises, blocks hunger and causes the thyroid to release thyroid hormones to increase metabolism. This allows you to achieve energy balance, known as homeostasis.

Generally speaking, people with lean body mass have low levels of leptin while obese people have higher levels of leptin. The fat cells release leptin to tell the brain how much body fat they carry. They tell the brain that there is plenty of fat stored, so eat less and burn more. Contrary, when we go awhile without eating, our fat stores go down and leptin goes down. Therefore, we eat more and burn less.

In obesity, there is a lot of body fat in their fat cells. Fat cells release leptin according to their size, so the more fat you have, the larger the leptin levels. The way this negative feedback loop works, these people should not be eating. The increased leptin levels from their full fat stores should be telling the brain to halt the consumption of food. The problem with obesity is that the leptin signal isn't working properly.

There is a ton of leptin floating around, but the brain is becoming unresponsive to the signal and is tricked into thinking there is too little leptin present. Your brain has essentially become numb to the "stop eating" warning.

This condition is known as leptin resistance. Leptin resistance develops in response to chronically elevated leptin levels. The brain eventually stops responding to the large amounts of leptin released, so you don't get the signal to stop eating. It mistakenly thinks the body is starving, even though it has more than enough fat stored. Therefore, the brain initiates two faulty changes in our physiology and behavior. First, it signals our body to eat more in order to not starve to death. Secondly, it reduces our metabolism (energy expenditure) because the brain thinks we need to conserve energy, making us burn fewer calories and making us feel sluggish and lazy.

FIGURE 9.2: LEPTIN RESISTANCE

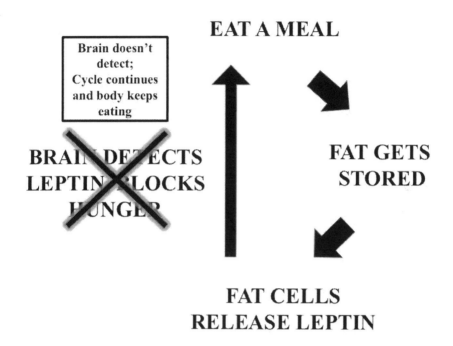

Remember the leptin thyroid connection? Normally high levels of leptin increase thyroid function to increase metabolism. In leptin resistance where the brain is numb to the excessive amounts of leptin, your thyroid goes into a fake starvation mode (aka leptin resistance). The hypothalamus can't sense the large amounts of leptin, so in turn the thyroid doesn't get properly turned on.

The thyroid then falsely sets its thyroid hormones on low metabolism mode in order to prevent the body from starving. Your brain mistakenly lowers your metabolism so you can survive a faulty famine, making weight loss nearly impossible and promoting weight gain instead. This leads to the body being drained of its energy, being tired all the time, and gaining weight. Sound familiar? This is very similar to insulin resistance discussed in the last chapter where your body eventually stops responding to chronically elevated insulin levels. The pancreas chronically produces large amounts of insulin in response to chronically elevated blood sugar, and the body fails to respond properly.

Another way of looking at it is leptin is part of your reward system. When you are healthy, leptin levels are low, and food becomes very rewarding when you are hungry. Leptin levels are raised after you eat. That is a signal that halts your potential reward system for food, so you don't need to keep on eating. This is why in normal conditions more food doesn't seem appetizing when you feel full.

Leptin resistance has a faulty reward system. This reward system doesn't adequately cue a person to halt eating when leptin rises. Leptin is being constantly produced in fat cells and is trying to tell the brain, "Stop eating!" The brain is unable to get the signal, so you feel hungrier and hungrier and the reward system doesn't get diminished. It becomes a vicious cycle, and leads to further obesity and chronic disease.

According to Dr. Guyenet, several cellular mechanisms can contribute to leptin resistance:

1. Inflammation: inflammation has been shown to give flawed signaling to the hypothalamus, likely contributing to leptin resistance.

2. Free Fatty Acids: elevated free fatty acids in the blood stream can impede with leptin signaling in the brain.

3. High Leptin Levels: having increased leptin levels initially can lead to a cascade reaction and stimulate leptin resistance.

All of the mentioned factors are increased in obesity. Once you are obese, this turns into a cycle that is hard to get out of. People get more and more obese as well as more leptin resistant over time.

So what is the solution to all of this? The good news is you can reset your leptin sensitivity! If you are overweight or obese, most likely you are leptin resistant. This is the case especially if you have excess fat in the mid-section. A big key to preventing and reversing leptin resistant is abiding by a diet that keeps inflammation and triglycerides low. Several things you can do right now is:

1. Avoid processed food: these kill the gut and increase inflammation

2. Consume healthy fats: healthy fats create building blocks for your hormones

3. Consume Soluble Fiber: improves gut health

4. Exercise: helps reverse leptin resistance

5. Sleep: poor sleep has negative effects on leptin. Not to mention the lack of energy you have to exercise, take care of yourself and make conscious, clear-headed decisions on a daily basis!

6. Reduce carbohydrate intake: helps lower blood triglycerides (free fatty acids) that interfere with leptin transport to the brain. This includes limiting / temporary eliminating sugar and fructose intake.

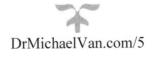

7. Healthy protein intake: improves leptin sensitivity

Did you notice anything about the above recommendations? You got it, these are the exact same guidelines for anyone wanting to be healthy, regardless of the circumstances. Eating real whole foods, keeping your gut healthy, daily exercise, and sleeping well are all lifestyle factors that contribute to health and wellness for life.

Where does intermittent fasting come into play here? Recent research out of the *International Journal of Obesity* found that intermittent fasting was affective at reducing leptin hormone and improving leptin resistance. In addition, it fights inflammation and lowers triglycerides.

Inflammation and high triglycerides are a few of the specific cellular mechanisms that actually cause leptin resistance in the first place. When you fast intermittently, body fat slowly comes off the body. Your body will naturally become lean over time and be able to maintain a low body fat set-point by steadily increasing leptin sensitivity (the opposite of leptin resistance).

Nutritional factors are very important here. It is critical to limit the amount of fructose and processed carbohydrates when resetting your leptin levels. Ideally, you should permanently limit processed carbohydrates for optimal health. Consuming healthy fats and protein will help you create building blocks for your hormones. These include healthy omega-3 fats, avocados, and high quality coconut oil. At the same time, you want to lower your omega-6 levels, which come from grains, conventional meats, and processed oils. Processed oils include grain derived oils and vegetable oils such as corn, soy, and canola. In addition, you also want to avoid unstable polyunsaturated oils like walnut, flax, and peanut oil. You will want to aim for getting 50-60% of calories from healthy fats, 20% from protein, and the rest from vegetables and fruits (more emphasis on vegetables).

Most people will start to experience weight loss and fat loss quickly, but some it can take a few weeks to get this whole process going. Be resilient! Your mood will improve and sleep quality will increase. Soon, energy levels will be increased, enough so you will actually want to exercise and still feel good after.

CHAPTER 10:

NORMALIZING GHRELIN LEVELS

Ghrelin is known as your body's hunger hormone. When you are running on an empty stomach, your stomach releases ghrelin. Ghrelin then sends a message to your hypothalamus in your brain telling you to eat. When you are full after a meal, ghrelin release is stopped, and your brain doesn't get a signal to keep eating. In normal situations, ghrelin levels are at their peak before eating and lowest about an hour after you've had a meal.

FIGURE 10.1: NORMAL GHRELIN FUNCTION

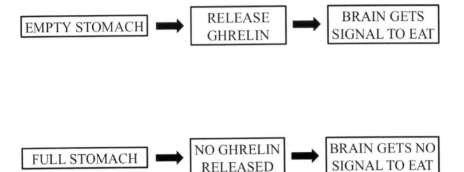

In overweight and obese people, however, fasting ghrelin levels are often lower than in people of normal weight. In addition, studies show that when overweight and obese people eat a meal, their ghrelin levels only decrease slightly. Under normal conditions, ghrelin levels should halt completely. This means that the hypothalamus doesn't receive as strong of a signal to stop eating, leading to overeating in many cases.

FIGURE 10.2: GHRELIN AND OBESITY

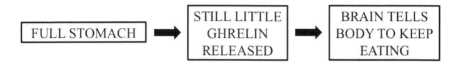

GLUCOSE VS FRUCTOSE

Many people say, "A calorie is a calorie," that it doesn't really matter whether you eat 100 calories of bread or 100 calories of broccoli because they have the same effect on your weight. This is a common lie that has been spread and has caused many people to count their calories instead of watching what foods they eat. It is true that calories have the same amount of energy, where one dietary calorie equals 4,184 Joules of energy; however, when it comes to your body and how it works, things are not that simple.

Our bodies are very complex biochemical systems. Different foods go through different biochemical pathways. Different foods have a major effect on the hormones and brain centers that control hunger and eating behavior.

For example, let's take a look at the sugars glucose and fructose. Glucose comes from starches like potatoes. Our bodies produce it and every cell in our body contains it. It is a molecule absolutely vital to life. Fructose, on the other hand, is the sugar from added sugars in many processed foods and is usually present in the form of high fructose corn syrup. We don't produce it and have never consumed it throughout evolutionary history except in the form of seasonally ripe fruits. The two seem almost identical, having the same chemical formula and weighing the exact same. To our body, however, the two are completely different. Sugar is not sugar.

Glucose can be metabolized by all of the tissues in our body, where fructose can only be metabolized by your liver. This is important and is part of the reason why fructose is so unhealthy. The entire burden of metabolizing fructose falls on your liver, which then promotes visceral fat. This is the harmful type of fat surrounding your organs in the abdominal area that is associated with a greater risk of heart disease. The metabolism of fructose by your liver creates a ton of waste products and toxins, including lots of uric acid, which increases your blood pressure and causes gout. Gout is a buildup of uric acid crystals in a joint leading to arthritis causing joint pain, swelling, heat and redness.

In contrast, every cell of your body, including your brain, utilizes glucose. Lots of the glucose you consume is burned immediately after you eat it. Fructose, on the other hand, turns into free fatty acids, VLDL (the worst type of cholesterol), and triglycerides, which get stored as fat. The free fatty acids created during fructose metabolism then get stored as fat droplets in your liver and skeletal muscle, causing insulin resistance and non-alcoholic fatty liver disease. Insulin resistance leads to metabolic syndrome, type II diabetes, and nearly every chronic disease out there. Under normal conditions, when you eat 120 calories of glucose, less than one calorie is stored as fat. When you eat 120 calories of fructose, nearly 40 of those calories are stored as fat.

Glucose suppresses the hunger hormone ghrelin and stimulates leptin, which will have the net effect of lowering or halting your appetite. What is interesting is that consuming fructose leads to higher ghrelin levels than glucose. In fact, fructose has actually been shown to have no effect on ghrelin levels. It also interferes with your brain's communication with leptin, resulting in overeating.

This means that consuming fructose gives you more of a tendency to eat way too much because the brain isn't getting the proper signals to stop eating. Fructose also doesn't stimulate the satiety centers in the brain the same way as glucose, leading to reduced satiety, leaving you feeling hungry and unsatisfied. This is why the consumption of fructose causes insulin resistance, increased belly fat, increased triglycerides, blood sugar, and small, dense LDL compared to the exact same number of calories from glucose.

FIGURE 10.3: GLUCOSE VS FRUCTOSE

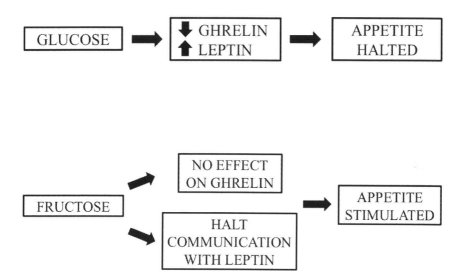

We are talking about the same number of calories, but vastly different effects in the body, including your hunger, hormones, and metabolic health. In truth, a calorie is NOT a calorie.

Now there is an important thing to keep in mind here. This applies only to fructose from added sugars. This doesn't include fructose from fruit, because fruits contain fiber, water, and significant chewing resistance that actually negate the negative effects from fructose. The bottom line is this. Even though fructose and glucose have the same structure, fructose has much more negative effects on hormones, appetite, and metabolic health.

By reducing processed carbohydrates in your diet and replacing them with high-quality fats and modest amounts of protein, you reduce ghrelin and boost several satiety hormones. These satiety hormones, or your appetite-reducing hormones, include glucagon-like peptide-1 (GLP-1), peptide YY, cholecystokinin, and leptin. This is why over 20 randomized controlled trials comparing low-carb and low-fat diets all come to the same conclusion: low carb diets lead to more weight loss. Not only do low-carb diets lead to drastically reduced appetites, but people start eating less calories without even trying because ghrelin, leptin, and insulin start to work the way they were designed.

Different sources of calories have vastly different effects on your hunger, hormones, energy expenditure, and the brain regions that control your food intake. Even though calories are important, they are not all made equal. Therefore, counting calories or even trying to be consciously aware of them is not necessary to get healthy and lose weight. In many cases, just simple changes in food selection and timing of your meals can lead to much better results.

INTERMITTENT FASTING AND GHRELIN

When ghrelin is present, we get hungry and most of us would head to the pantry for a snack or a meal. This meal would then decrease ghrelin, and therefore would relieve our hunger. By doing so, however, we miss out on many of the benefits that ghrelin can offer, such as its potent ability to stimulate growth hormone. What this means is that when you eat less frequently and allow larger amounts of ghrelin to be present in your body, you can effectively raise your growth hormone levels. To take advantage of this growth hormone spike, it is important to also exercise while ghrelin levels are high, spiking growth hormone even more.

FIGURE 10.4: INTERMITTENT FASTING'S EFFECT ON GHRELIN

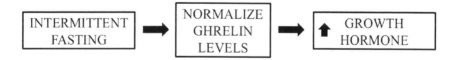

On the contrary, remember when I said that obese people have lower fasting levels of ghrelin? When ghrelin is present in your body in lower amounts, growth hormone will not be effectively released. Therefore, people with obesity won't get proper amounts of this "fitness hormone" that allows your body to look young and vibrant and have a healthy amount of muscle mass throughout life.

FIGURE 10.5: OBESITY AND GHRELIN

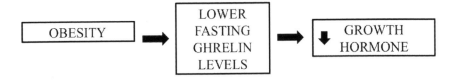

The brain also benefits from ghrelin being present in the body and fighting the urge to eat all day. In fact, studies have shown that ghrelin can have positive effects on learning and memory, and that learning may be best during the day when ghrelin levels are high.

FIGURE 10.6: GHRELIN'S EFFECT ON LEARNING AND MEMORY

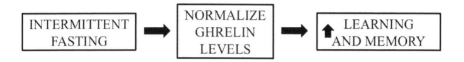

To properly take advantage of ghrelin, you need to adopt an intermittent fasting regimen and eat less frequently. As I mentioned earlier, I would advise to work out in a fasted state, preferably before your first meal of the day. This will allow you to workout when ghrelin levels are at its peak, taking advantage of the elevated growth hormone levels. This will also help maximally replenish your body and muscles when you enjoy your first big meal immediately after your workout. See Chapter 7 on your mTOR pathway for more information on how to maximize your workout and the proper post workout meal to best increase muscle mass.

It turns out that breakfast, the supposed most important meal of the day, actually starts your day off by decreasing ghrelin. This sabotages your goal of better health and physique. Furthermore, by suppressing ghrelin with frequent meals starting with breakfast, you are missing out on the elevated ability to learn, retain the information you learn and provide an effective defense against the effects of stress. Once you retrain your body to NOT expect food all day, or in this case the first thing in the morning, these side effects of hunger become less of an issue due to the normalizing of your ghrelin levels. Therefore, an easy solution to normalizing ghrelin levels and getting all the benefits it comes with is as simple as postponing your first meal of the day.

FIGURE 10.7: GHRELIN'S EFFECT ON HUNGER

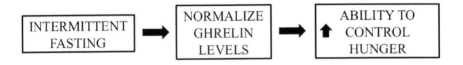

Think of our ancestors. They likely needed elevated ghrelin levels, and the subsequent increase in growth hormone, mental alertness, etc. in order to hunt and kill their pray. If we adopt this same template of eating in today's world, we can utilize ghrelin not to track down wild animals, but to utilize the benefits each day at work and in our exercise routine.

Your body's level of ghrelin is also influenced by other factors, including your lifestyle habits. For example, lack of sleep increases ghrelin, making you feel hungry when you shouldn't be. Have you ever experienced the should-I-go-to-bed-or-have-a-midnight-snack conundrum? This a major reason why a lack of sleep is linked to weight gain. Stress, anger, sadness, and other negative emotions also alter these hunger hormones, which is why most people experiencing these emotions seek food as a coping mechanism.

CHAPTER 11:

INFLAMMATION

Inflammation is the body's normal process of repairing damaged tissue and protecting itself from foreign invaders like bacteria and viruses. In fact, we need a certain level of inflammation to be healthy. The issue here is understanding the difference between chronic and acute inflammation.

Acute inflammation is absolutely necessary to help protect and heal the body from an injury or infection. By a series of complex reactions, your body's immune system sends out white blood cells and other chemicals to the injured areas to fight off potentially harmful foreign bodies. If you have ever gotten a cut or an infection, then you have certainly experienced this beneficially acute inflammatory process. Symptoms include:

- Redness

- Warmth

- Pain

- Swelling

- Loss of movement

- Loss of function

When the inflammation becomes chronic, there are usually no symptoms that occur until you experience a loss of function. Chronic inflammation is a slow and systemic process that silently damages your tissues until you notice the major result of a disease process. This process can persist for years until you are finally diagnosed with something significant like heart disease, cancer, or Alzheimer's disease.

A wide range of health problems, including, but not limited to, heart disease, stroke, obesity, migraines, cancer, chronic pain, thyroid issues, diabetes, dental issues, ADD/ADHD, peripheral neuropathy, and autoimmune diseases like multiple sclerosis, ulcerative colitis, Crohn's disease, and rheumatoid arthritis are all rooted in chronic inflammation. In fact, you could argue that without chronic inflammation, almost all diseases around the world would not even exist. This excessive amount of inflammation must be properly addressed if you wish to be healed.

FIGURE 11.1: CHRONIC INFLAMMATION

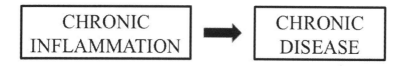

Chronic inflammation is caused largely by an unhealthy lifestyle. It is the result of a mal-functioning or over-reactive immune system, or an underlying problem that the body is trying to fight. Things that increase this harmful type of inflammation include chronically eating an unhealthy omega-3 to omega-6 ratio and consuming too much sugar. Omega-6 fatty acids are inflammatory, while healthy omega-3 fatty acids are anti-inflammatory. In order to help reduce chronic inflammation, we should consume healthy fats like animal-based omega-

3 fats or the essential fatty acids gamma linolenic acid (GLA) and conjugated linolenic acid (CLA) found in grass-fed meats.

All of the following can increase your risk of chronic inflammation:

- Being overweight and / or obese

- Consuming a poor diet (like mentioned above)

- Sedentary lifestyle

- Stress

What is sad is that many are suffering from many of the above disorders, but have absolutely no idea on how to eliminate the inflammation. Most doctors out there are using pharmaceutical drugs in an attempt to get to the root cause, only to find excessive side effects and sickness as a result. If you know that drugs for inflammation down regulate the immune system, that they do not stop the underlying disease process, and that they do not allow the damaged tissues in the body to regenerate, why would anyone go that route?

Unless you cease the actual cause of the inflammatory response, all you have really done by taking anti-inflammatory drugs is postpone the inevitable by continuing to destroy the body even more during the process. We see ads on TV everyday showing how pharmaceutical drug companies are hiring big named spokespeople to adopt and promote their product. These drugs mask the inflammation and suppress the immune system. None of these drugs have the ability to correct the underlying problem, yet the imagery of the drug ads gives viewers the false hope that they can, indeed, get their life back.

To test for chronic inflammation, usually conventional medicine recommends the C-reactive protein (CRP) test. This measures a certain protein in the body that is made by the liver and released into the bloodstream in response to a tissue injury, the start of an infection, or some other cause of inflammation. A high level of CRP in the blood is a sign that there may be an inflammatory process occurring in the body.

Other markers of inflammation include an increase in the ESR (erythrocyte sedimentation rate), fasting blood insulin levels, and tumor necrosis factor-alpha (TNF-α). TNF-α seems to be increased in obese subjects, suggesting its role as a pro-inflammatory protein in response to insulin resistance and metabolic abnormalities. TNF-α, being a potent marker of inflammation, has been linked to a decrease in the number of neural stem cells and a decrease in the brain's ability to make new cells.

INTERMITTENT FASTING AND INFLAMMATION

A decrease in the level of BDNF (brain derived neurotrophic factor) is also a sign of an inflammatory process in the body. Exercise and intermittent fasting have been proven to reduce inflammation in the body and improve brain function by increasing BDNF, allowing old nerve cells to form dense, interconnected webs that make the brain run faster and more efficiently. BDNF allows the process of neuroplasticity to take place, which describes the brain's dynamic ability to reorganize itself by forming new neural connections and to form new brain cells throughout life.

BDNF and inflammation in the brain are indirectly related, so BDNF can only increase in the brain when inflammation levels are low. Therefore, the more that BDNF assembles in the brain from incorporating intermittent fasting, the lower amount of inflammation present. It also increases blood and oxygen flow to the brain, and actually can increase the size of the frontal lobes. The frontal lobes, located at the front of the brain, is the part of the brain that controls important cognitive skills in humans, such as emotional expression, problem solving, memory, language, judgment, and sexual behavior.

FIGURE 11.2: THE EFFECTS OF CHRONIC INFLAMMATION

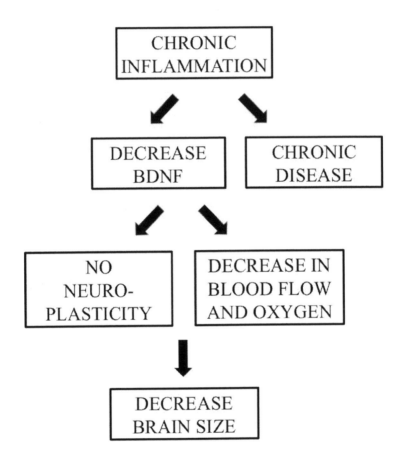

The hippocampus is one of the areas of the brain that BDNF acts on. BDNF actually stimulates the production of new brain cells here in response to intermittent fasting. In contrast, we also know that the hippocampus is negatively stimulated by stress and inflammation. The consequences of inflammation on the brain's ability to make new cells is extreme. It diminishes the survival rate of previously existing neurons / brain cells and inhibits the brain's ability to make new neurons. It also has implications on cognition, resulting in a decrease in memory and compromises the ability to learn new things.

For example, tumor necrosis factor—alpha (TNF-α) is a potent marker of inflammation. TNF-α has been linked to a decrease in the number of neural stem cells, a decrease in the brain's ability to make new cells, and an increase in the degenerative processes in the brain.

Mark Mattson, senior investigator for the National Institute on Aging, did a study on overweight adults with moderate asthma. By reducing their caloric intake by 80% every other day for eight weeks, they were able to reduce their body weight by eight percent, as well as reduce markers of oxidative stress and inflammation. Asthma-related symptoms improved as well, along with several quality-of-life indicators.

Mattson and his colleagues did a separate 2011 study out of the *International Journal of Obesity* and found that intermittent fasting was effective at reducing free androgen index, high-sensitivity C-reactive protein, total and LDL cholesterol, triglycerides, blood pressure, and increasing sex hormone binding globulin and IGF binding proteins 1 and 2. All of those substances serve as potent markers of inflammation that are devastating to one's health. The research really shows how powerful intermittent fasting can be at combating this stressful environment and getting to the bottom of this inflammatory disaster.

Another study out of the journal *Free Radical Biology and Medicine* also revealed that oxidative stress and inflammation declined in response to intermittent fasting. These findings demonstrated rapid and sustained beneficial effects of intermittent fasting on the underlying disease processes.

One of my favorite studies that was analyzed looked at Muslim individuals following Ramadan intermittent fasting (RIF) in the journal *Nutritional Research*. Ramadan is a holy month in the Islamic calendar, where Muslims must abstain from eating or drinking during daylight hours. This results in approximately 12 hours of fasting each day, giving us one of the more natural models to study the intermittent fasting effects in humans. Proinflammatory proteins, including tumor necrosis

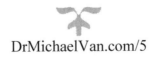

factor α, systolic and diastolic blood pressures, body weight, and body fat percentage were significantly lower during Ramadan as compared with the same subjects before Ramadan started. The conclusion was:

> *"These results indicate that RIF attenuates inflammatory status of the body by suppressing proinflammatory cytokine expression and decreasing body fat and circulating levels of leukocytes."*

Wow, that is a lot of science. To simplify everything, chronic inflammation and oxidative stress is bad for the body and leads to obesity and many chronic diseases. It increases inflammatory proteins in the brain that lead to the breaking down of brain cells as well as blocking the brain's ability to make new, healthy cells. It decreases BDNF, the substance that activates new brain stem cells and gives the brain lots of protection.

The best news of all is that intermittent fasting has been proven to decrease inflammation, thereby preventing chronic disease. As stated before, it increases BDNF in the brain, enhancing neuroplasticity, and produces blood flow and oxygenation. As a result, intermittent fasting has shown the ability to increase the size of your brain. Wow! Show me anything other intervention that can do this besides exercise. There isn't one, so don't waste your time.

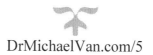

FIGURE 11.3: FASTING AND INFLAMMATION

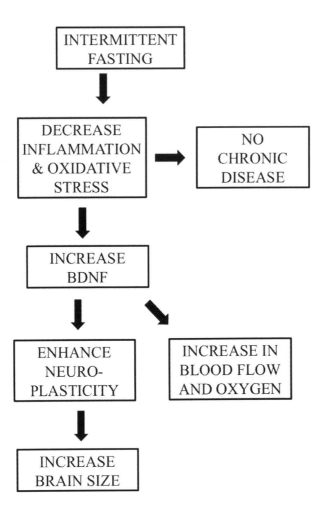

CHAPTER 12:

HEART HEALTH

By now, we already know that intermittent fasting can help with heart health in a number of ways. We learned from previous chapters how it can reduce chronic inflammation and improve insulin sensitivity, preventing all chronic diseases like heart disease. In fact, increasing insulin sensitivity can reduce your risk of heart disease by 93%! We know that it is effective at reducing visceral fat, the harmful type of fat surrounding your organs in the abdominal area that is associated with a greater risk of heart disease. We know that many disease processes originate in the digestive system and that intermittent fasting helps to optimize the bacteria in the gut promoting health and longevity. We also know that our body, including the heart and muscles, operate very efficiently when they get the majority of their energy via ketones, drastically improving immune and heart function.

When dealing specifically with the heart, many experts look at factors such as cholesterol levels, triglycerides, blood pressure, and inflammatory markers. It just so happens that intermittent fasting is quite exceptional at reducing these risk factors. It has been established that intermittent fasting reduces LDL cholesterol, blood triglycerides, inflammatory markers, blood sugar and insulin resistance. These are all major risk factors for heart disease, the number one cause of death in the world.

In a study out of *The Journal of Nutritional Biochemistry*, Mattson noted that intermittent fasting (IF) and caloric restriction (CR):

> *"Enhance cardiovascular and brain functions and improve several risk factors for coronary artery disease and stroke including a reduction in blood pressure and increased insulin sensitivity. Cardiovascular stress adaptation is improved and heart rate variability is increased."*

In addition, Mattson stated that subjects:

"Maintained on an IF regimen exhibit increased resistance of heart and brain cells to ischemic injury in experimental models of myocardial infarction and stroke. The beneficial effects of IF and CR result from at least two mechanisms — reduced oxidative damage and increased cellular stress resistance."

FIGURE 12.1: INTERMITTENT FASTING'S ABILITY AT REDUCING RISK FACTORS FOR HEART DISEASE

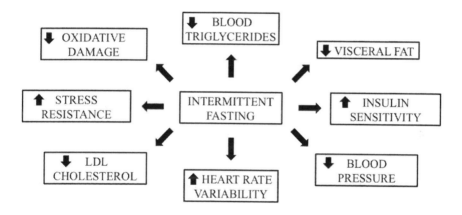

There you have it. As the language can get a little complex in journal articles, let me describe this to you in layman's terms. This study talks about intermittent fasting and how it allows the brain and heart to be resistant to ischemic injury. Ischemic injury is a restriction in blood supply to tissues, causing a shortage of oxygen and glucose for cellular metabolism that is needed to keep tissues and cells alive.

Oxygen is carried to tissues of the body from the blood, so insufficient blood supply causes the tissue to become depleted of oxygen. The brain and heart are very aerobic, meaning they require a ton of oxygen in order to generate energy. What is interesting (and scary) is that in as little as 3-4 minutes of limited blood flow, the brain and heart can suffer irreversible damage. This contrasts with other tissues in the body, which can take up to 20 minutes of decreased blood flow to get the same damaging effect.

Insufficient blood flow to the heart is caused by a condition known as atherosclerosis, where you get accumulation of cholesterol and fatty-rich plaques in the arteries. If arteries carrying blood to the heart become blocked from these hardened plaques, the heart muscle will receive less oxygen and start to die off rapidly. This results in ischemic heart disease, the most common cause of death in the Western world. Since the heart and brain need lots of oxygen and glucose for energy, preventing any type of ischemic injury by promoting blood flow, oxygen, and energy exchange is very important. Intermittent fasting, exercise, and proper nutrition does just that.

It is important to take a moment and discuss the mechanism of artery damage here. Saying that there is an accumulation of cholesterol and fatty-rich plaques may lead you to think that cholesterol and fat are the cause, which they are NOT. In fact, understanding this point can actually make you more educated than 99% of the doctors out there who try and blame cholesterol for everything in order to increase cholesterol-lowering drug profits.

What actually causes atherosclerosis is damage to the inner layer of blood vessels. These become damaged by a chronic stressful lifestyle. Let me explain.

A chronic stressful lifestyle usually includes something like this: Working overtime, constantly working at the computer, stressed to meet deadlines, slamming down energy drinks and coffee for energy, not moving or exercising, eating processed non-fiber carbohydrates in the form of refined sugar and high fructose corn syrup and fats in the form of trans fats or hydrogenated fats with chemical colors and preservatives.

Does this sound familiar to anyone? This chronic stressful lifestyle actually damages the endothelium of the blood vessels.

Exercise, for example, produces nitric oxide in our blood vessels. Nitric oxide helps the vessels relax and open up in diameter in order to carry more blood flow. This process is called vasodilation. High levels of nitric oxide production are important in protecting organs such as the heart and brain from ischemic damage. With a lack of exercise and movement, that means there is also a lack of nitric oxide opening up the arteries. This combined with a poor diet actually damages the endothelium of the blood vessels, causing an inflammatory response. The chronic destructive lifestyle is the cause.

This process of arterial damage leads to an increase in cholesterol being released from the liver and into the bloodstream to the site of tissue damage. Cholesterol has an important role in repairing damaged tissue in the body. In this case, the cholesterol is needed to repair the tissue damage caused by this destructive lifestyle. This process also recruits white blood cells to the area to fight against the inflammation and heal the damage. The result is regrowth of the inner lining of the blood vessel around the damage, leading to a blood vessel with a smaller diameter. This makes it more likely for ischemia to take place because there is a smaller diameter, which means less oxygen transfer.

FIGURE 12.2: MECHANISM OF ARTERIAL DAMAGE

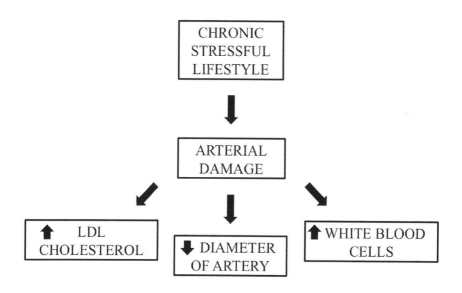

Here is the question: if excessive damage to the arteries from a poor lifestyle occurs, making it necessary to distribute extra cholesterol through the bloodstream, would it seem very wise to merely lower the cholesterol artificially with a drug and forget about why it is elevated in the first place? Wouldn't it seem much smarter to instead reduce the need for the extra cholesterol, which is the poor lifestyle causing the

damage? The increase in cholesterol and clotting factors in the form of
white blood cells is an intelligent response to repair arterial damage. It
doesn't matter what drug you take in this condition, if you don't escape
that unhealthy lifestyle, it's over.

Sure, you can take a drug to lower cholesterol. You can take a
drug to lower heart rate and blood pressure in the form of a beta blocker.
You can take a drug to thin the blood, a drug to lower blood sugar. You
can even do a randomized controlled trial to prove that a cholesterol
lowering drug can indeed lower cholesterol. However, you will never
find a study that says it makes you healthier or increases life span. Why
can't you find a study showing these pharmaceutical drugs increase
lifespan and health? Because they don't exist!

What does exist is a new study out of the journal *Expert Review
of Clinical Pharmacology* called, "Statins stimulate atherosclerosis and
heart failure: pharmacological mechanisms." Yes, you read that
correctly. In contrast to the current belief that cholesterol reduction with
drugs decreases atherosclerosis, it is actually shown they do just the
opposite. They cause coronary artery calcification and impair muscle
function in the heart and blood vessels. We have all been fooled. Even
with these studies coming out, cholesterol-lowering drugs are the most
commonly prescribed medication in the United States. Sales continue to

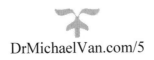

skyrocket on the market and bring in billions of dollars every year. What a scam!

In the meantime, the person taking cholesterol-lowering drugs (statins) is still sick and dying. They will just die without high cholesterol with no extra days added to their life. Worse of all, pharmaceuticals do not encourage the patient to maintain a healthy lifestyle now that they have a makeshift remedy, like a band aide on a gapping wound. Sounds scientific to me. Why not implement lifestyle factors that are actually proven to prevent this whole process from taking place, such as diet, exercise, and intermittent fasting?

My vision for the future of healthcare would involve a doctor telling this to a sick patient, something I personally tell patients on a daily basis: "I want you to meditate for 20 minutes a day, exercise for at least 20-30 minutes a day, apply intermittent fasting, avoid processed foods, eat plenty of organic vegetables and fruit, spend more time in nature and less indoors, stop worrying about things you can't control and ditch your T.V. Come back in 3 weeks." If you have a doctor who pushes medications over lifestyle changes, you may need to re-evaluate your situation. As my favorite saying goes, "The sign of a good doctor should be how many patients he can get OFF medications, not how many people he puts ON medications."

Another interesting study from the journal *Annals of Nutrition and Metabolism* evaluated the change in cardiovascular health in Muslim individuals before and after Ramadan. The results showed significant improvements in their lipid profile. HDL levels increased and the Total Cholesterol/HDL Cholesterol ratio decreased, a ratio that is commonly used to predict ischemic heart disease. In addition, it decreased levels of the D-dimer test, which means that the blood is less likely to form inappropriate blood clots, similarly to what happens in cases of stroke. It also reduced homocysteine levels, where high levels are associated with atherosclerosis and blood clots. This all translates to an improved blood coagulation profile. It means that the blood is able to form a clot when necessary, like when repairing a damaged vessel. It also prevents the harmful type of clotting that can produce damage in the body and lead to ischemic heart disease. The level of CRP was also decreased. CRP rises when there is harmful inflammation throughout the body and is helpful in determining the potential risk level for cardiovascular disease, heart attacks, and strokes.

Finally, a separate study out of the *American Journal of Clinical Nutrition* analyzed intermittent fasting's effect on body weight and heart disease risk factors in obese adults. Sixteen obese subjects were used and put on an intermittent fasting regimen for 10 weeks. What they discovered was yet another promising finding, supporting the efficacy of intermittent fasting's positive health benefits, specifically on the heart.

These results included weight loss and a reduction in fat tissue mass, blood pressure, and heart rate. There was a significant improvement in lipid profile, with a decrease in total cholesterol and LDL-cholesterol and an increase in HDL-cholesterol. Specifically, the percentage of body fat in the subjects of this study decreased by an average of 3% and systolic blood pressure was lowered by an average of 8 mm Hg. The conclusion of the study suggested that intermittent fasting is a:

> "viable diet option to help obese individuals lose weight and decrease CAD risk."

This all happened during 10 weeks of intermittent fasting every other day. These amazing results all came without subjects incorporating an exercise program, so think of what the benefits could have been if both were combined! Again, try and find any other lifestyle intervention that can do this besides a specific exercise plan. Like I always say, they don't exist so don't waste your time.

Harmful lifestyle factors are the number one contribution to the development of cardiovascular disease, the leading cause of death worldwide. Traditional approaches of treatment have been proven ineffective in most people; however, intermittent fasting has shown to have a positive impact on heart health and in the prevention of such risk factors. It has been shown effective against inflammation and oxidative stress, resulting in the prevention and the reversal of atherosclerosis. If you are looking for a lifestyle intervention that is researched and shows undeniable results for the prevention of heart disease, look no further than intermittent fasting.

CHAPTER 13:

OXIDATIVE STRESS &

FREE RADICAL DAMAGE

Aging is known to be associated with in increased amount of reactive oxygen species (ROS), which are a fancy name for free radicals. When we age, we slowly build up an accumulation of free radicals that are responsible for the slow damaging of our DNA and proteins in the body. Studies show that there is a clear direct correlation between the amount of oxidative stress (free radical damage) and the effects of aging. Antioxidants are molecules that prevent or delay cell damage by inhibiting the oxidation process. When you are deficient in antioxidant defenses, oxidative stress accumulates in our body and leads to advanced aging. The more we can keep our antioxidant system intact, the more

we can negate oxidative stress accumulation and delay the aging
process.

Remember when we discussed the role of free radicals and
antioxidants in the lifespan and longevity chapter? One of the main
reasons intermittent fasting has such a powerful effect on reducing free
radical damage is its ability to promote fat burning in the body. Burning
fat as our primary fuel is a lot cleaner than burning carbohydrates
because fat burning generates far less free radicals. Glucose is known as
a more "dirty" type of fuel because it produces a lot more reactive
oxygen species that damage DNA and can increase the likelihood for
illness and disease to develop.

One way to combat this free radical damage is to provide your
body an adequate defense against them in the form of antioxidants.
These antioxidants include glutathione, vitamin C, resveratrol,
carotenoids, astaxanthin, CoQ10, alpha-lipoic acid, and vitamin E. As
long as you consume a balanced, unprocessed diet full of high-quality
raw organic vegetables and fruits, your body will acquire these essential
antioxidants naturally. You will also achieve greater amounts of
beneficial antioxidant levels with intermittent fasting.

Another way to give your body protection against oxidative damage is to avoid or reduce the excessive accumulation of free radical damage in the first place. Intermittent fasting does just that by allowing the body to burn a clean fuel like fat instead of relying solely on the dirty fuel in the form of excessive carbs.

In the journal *Mechanisms of Ageing and Development*, they showed that intermittent fasting for four months significantly reduced oxidative stress and free radical damage. This study revealed that intermittent fasting exerted this benefit by significantly decreasing free radical formation, giving the body's cells a positive antioxidant effect that effectively decreased oxidation and DNA damage.

The benefits here stem from increasing the efficiency of the mitochondria, known as the powerhouses of the cell. Mitochondria are kind of like the digestive system where they are responsible for taking in nutrients, breaking them down, and creating energy-rich molecules for our cells. They are the working structures in the cell that keeps the cell full of energy.

In normal conditions of the mitochondria, there is a balance between antioxidant protection and free radicals. These free radicals are maintained at non-toxic levels due to the presence of antioxidants as well as repair enzymes. By reducing free radicals, intermittent fasting effectively reduces the likelihood of various pathological processes that cause tissue damage and cell death.

Mark Mattson, senior investigator for the National Institute on Aging, did a study on overweight adults with moderate asthma and found similar results. By reducing their caloric intake by 80% every other day for eight weeks (alternate day intermittent fasting), they were able to reduce their body weight by eight percent, as well as reduce markers of oxidative stress and inflammation. This study brings to light that intermittent fasting counteracts disease processes in the body by promoting less free radical accumulation as well as reduced inflammation. In addition, asthma-related symptoms improved, along with several quality-of-life indicators.

We know that oxidative stress plays a major role in not just the ageing process, but in the diseases most commonly responsible for mortality. We also know that intermittent fasting reduces oxidative damage by actually reducing free radical accumulation in the body. Controlled studies have even shown that intermittent fasting increases the resistance of cells to various types of stress. For example, the mortality from natural causes or mortality caused by oxidative stress is significantly reduced in animals maintaining an intermittent fasting regimen compared to control animals consuming a normal diet.

What scientists are also finding is that intermittent fasting results in a huge accumulation of antioxidants and protective proteins in the body. For example, subjects maintained on an intermittent fasting regimen exhibit greater amounts of the antioxidants vitamin E and coenzyme Q10. They also have higher plasma membrane redox enzyme activities in brain cells compared to subjects being fed ad libitum (eating freely; no restrictions). Intermittent fasting actually activates the expression of proteins involved in the regulation of cellular energy. These energy pathways include mitochondrial oxidative phosphorylation, glycolysis, and our NAD/NADH metabolism. Our energy production pathways are enhanced by intermittent fasting, turning ourselves into efficient energy-producing machines.

In addition, intermittent fasting increases the levels of heat-shock proteins that protect crucial proteins in the body against damage. These specific protective proteins include HSP-70 in liver cells as well as glucose-regulated protein 78 in the brain. The name of these compounds are not important, but the increased protection they give to the body are.

DrMichaelVan.com/5

The bottom line is this: intermittent fasting both increases our antioxidant defenses in our body as well as reducing free radical damage. The end result is a more efficient human body with increased cellular protection to adequately thrive in this world we live in.

FIGURE 13.1: INTERMITTENT FASTING AND OXIDATIVE STRESS

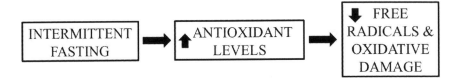

CHAPTER 14:

CANCER

Imagine there was a commercial plane crash causing many deaths. A major plane crash, no doubt, would make headlines on news channels everywhere. Now imagine there was nearly 8-10 of these plane crashes every day killing everyone on board. This massive amount of deaths is the equivalent to how many people die from cancer each and every day.

When you dig deeper, the statistics do not get any prettier. Two million Americans are diagnosed with cancer every year. One person out of three will be diagnosed with cancer at some point in their lives.

- In the early 1900's, 1 in 20 people developed cancer

- In the 1940's, 1 in 16 people developed cancer

- In the 1970's, 1 in 10 people developed cancer

- Today, a whopping 1 in 3 develop cancer!

Here is what we do know. These figures and statistics are occurring in spite of the massive technological advances we have made in the last 50 years. Western medicine is no closer to finding a cancer cure now than it was back then. The only consistent thing with these technological advances over the last half century is that the worldwide epidemic of cancer is growing in staggering proportions.

With these statistics, the likelihood is high that many of you reading this book either have cancer now, have previously had it, or have loved ones that have cancer. What you need to understand is that cancer is a big business bringing in billions of dollars a year. The sad part is that virtually none of this money is being spent on effective cancer prevention strategies. This includes dietary guidelines, exercise and obesity education. What this industry is doing instead is pouring out its money into treating cancer, not preventing or curing it.

On average, the typical cancer patient will spend around $50,000 fighting the disease. Chemotherapy drugs just happen to be the most expensive treatments on the market. If Big Pharma can keep the money-making machine running, then they can continue to make huge profits on chemotherapy drugs, radiotherapy, diagnostic procedures, and surgeries.

Even with the massive amounts of money being put into cancer research, still two out of every three cancer patients will pass away/lose their battle within five years after receiving their standard treatment – surgery, radiation, and chemotherapy. Even being conservative, chemotherapy benefits about 1 out of every 20 people with cancer.

Does it even make sense that two of these three 'treatments' are carcinogenic themselves?! For example, a mammogram, the conventional go-to "prevention" strategy for breast cancer, is pushed on females once they hit their 40's and 50's. They want you to get them annually in hope that they can detect the cancer earlier with the purpose of starting the expensive trifecta of treatment earlier. The problem? According to the Institute of Medicine, they emit 1000x the amount of radiation compared to a standard chest x-ray. Does it seem ironic that females will radiate their breasts year after year for decades even though the medical professionals giving this advice know that ionizing radiation causes cancer? Radiation induced cancer is dose-responsive, so the greater the dose, the higher the risk of cancer developing.

The other problem with mammograms? They are one of the most useless, unreliable medical screenings around today. Researchers at the *Nordic Cochrane Center in Denmark* studied 600,000 healthy women. This is what they found:

If 2000 women are screened with mammograms regularly for 10 years:

- One will benefit from screening, as she will avoid dying from breast cancer because the screening detected the cancer earlier.

- 200 healthy women will experience a false alarm. 10 of those 200 will have either part of their breast or the whole breast removed, and they will often receive radiation, and most likely, chemotherapy.

Still not convinced? Check out these findings from other studies:

- In the *Journal of the American Medical Association,* Harvard and Dartmouth analyzed 10 years' worth of mammogram screenings, breast cancer diagnoses and deaths from 550 counties across America involving 16 million women. Conclusion: no evidence that getting a mammogram will add a day to your life.

- From the *British Medical Journal* and as reported by the *New York Times*, one of the largest and longest studies of mammography to date, involving 90,000 women followed for 25 years in Canada, found that mammograms have absolutely NO impact on breast cancer mortality.

- According to the *Cochrane Database*, mammograms do not reduce the overall risk of dying, or the overall risk of dying from cancer. Women who get their recommended frequency of mammograms do not live longer than women who do not get mammograms.

Again, the cancer industry has been spreading misinformation to the public so we can get the perception that they have been actively seeking a cure for many years. The truth? The cancer epidemic is an absolute dream for Big Pharma, and their campaigns to silence proven cancer cures have been wildly aggressive. Just watch the documentary film, *"Cancer: Forbidden Cures."*

Think about it, what would happen if the cancer industry allowed a cure? Boom, in an instant their patient base goes away. Financially, (and maliciously I might add) it makes more sense to keep the huge abundance of cancer patients alive, sick, and coming back for more. Well guess what, that is exactly what is happening.

Just look into Dr. Burzynski and the Burzynski Clinic. This brave doctor and scientist invented some of the best cancer treatments and cures in the world, backed with randomized controlled clinical trials. This seems like great news, but there is one problem. The FDA is trying to stand in his way and block these treatments from being used and put on the market. If this happened, it would mark the first time in history a single scientist, not a pharmaceutical company, would hold the exclusive patent and distribution rights on a paradigm-shifting medical breakthrough. And Big Pharma can't let that happen.

His treatments are responsible for curing some of the most incurable forms of terminal cancer without the use of any surgery, chemotherapy, or radiation. Dr. Burzynski went through a treacherous, 14-year battle to obtain FDA-approval, and when you look into the facts of this story, you will never look at our healthcare system and the FDA the same again. They even tried him at the state supreme court to halt his practices and engaged in four Federal Grand Juries spanning over a decade, all of which ended up finding no fault on his behalf. Can you say conflict of interest?

Finally, he was indicted in their 5th Grand Jury in 1995, resulting in two federal trials and two sets of jurors finding him not guilty of any wrongdoing. If he was convicted, he could have faced 290 years in federal prison and $18.5 million in fines. The guy cured cancer safely and effectively! Isn't that what the Food and Drug Administration would want? I guess it is wishful thinking on my part.

This is just one of the several natural treatments out there that have been used successfully to treat cancer. Of course, all of these treatments have been violently discounted, silenced, and pushed under the radar by the medical monopoly. Not to mention the smearing, jailing, and the professional ruining of these physicians' and researchers' careers who made these brilliant and ground-breaking discoveries. All this for daring to question and confront the medical establishment. In order to keep the medical monopoly protected, any effective natural treatment is met with massive opposition by the pharmaceutical and medical industries. They have proven time and time again that they are willing to go to extreme measures to prevent the truth from reaching the public. If they cannot patent the treatment, it gets in the way of their revenue. The FDA is now primarily funded by the drug companies, restricting competition and protecting the profits.

It isn't all bad news. There are many steps you can take to lower your risk of cancer, but you have to take preventative steps immediately. It makes much more sense to get healthy and prevent cancer from occurring in the first place than to treat it. I truly believe you can virtually eliminate the risk of cancer and chronic disease by changing your lifestyle to one that is genetically congruent for health and vitality.

KETOGENIC DIET & INTERMITTENT FASTING

To expand on the above list, I think the most powerful strategy out there to avoid or treat cancer is to starve your cancer cells by depriving them of their only food source – sugar. Normal cells in your body can adapt to different energy sources, allowing them to use both carbs and fat for fuel. Cancer cells, on the other hand, do not express that metabolic flexibility and are only able to use sugar as an energy source. A man by the name of Dr. Otto Warburg was actually given the Nobel Prize in Physiology for this discovery over 75 years ago, and still virtually no oncologist actually uses this information! He discovered that cancer cells have a fundamentally different energy metabolism compared to healthy cells. He called his theory the "Warburg Effect," which occurs in up to 80 percent of cancers.

THE SCIENTIFIC APPROACH TO
INTERMITTENT FASTING

FIGURE 14.1: NORMAL CELLS VS CANCER CELLS

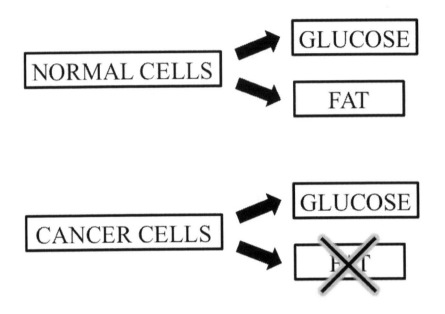

Later, analysis from PET scans revealed cancer was found in places in the body where cells consume the most glucose (sugar). In fact, the more glucose a tumor consumes, the worst a patient's prognosis. Unfortunately, Dr. Warburg's work vanished for many decades because of scientists shifting their attention to genetics. Now they realized that it's not the genetic defects that cause cancer. Rather, mitochondrial damage happens first, which then triggers nuclear genetic mutations in the DNA. Unbelievable!

Depriving your body of sugar by incorporating a ketogenic diet, especially when combined with hyperbaric oxygen therapy, is highly recommended as it will starve cancer cells. As said from Thomas Seyfried, Ph.D., who is the leader in treating cancer nutritionally:

> *"Calorie restriction and restricted ketogenic diets, which reduce circulating glucose levels and elevate ketone levels, are anti-invasive, anti antiogenic, and pro-apoptotic towards malignant brain cancer."*

Carbs turn into glucose in the body. Cancer cells need glucose to thrive. Cutting carbs from your diet reduces glucose levels in the blood, therefore literally starving your cancer cells. Interestingly, even Metformin, a drug used in the treatment of diabetes that reduces blood glucose levels, also has been proven to reduce cancer. Even though, like all drugs, it causes a ton of harmful side effects, it still illustrates the point that by reducing blood sugar levels, you reduce and can even reverse cancer.

FIGURE 14.2: KETOGENIC DIET AND CANCER

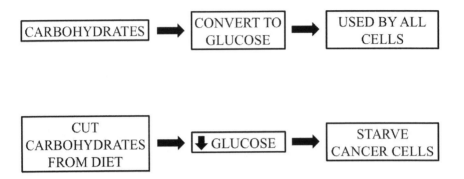

Then there is intermittent fasting. Would you believe me if I told you that not only can intermittent fasting enhance the lifespan of those with cancer, but it can also work to prevent cancer from occurring in the first place? This is exactly what the available evidence on the subject matter tells us.

Let's look at those already with cancer. There was a study in the journal called *Cancer Investigation* where they took two groups of rats. In one group, they put them on an intermittent fasting regimen, and in the other group, they allowed them to eat freely (ad libitum) whenever they wanted and whatever they wanted. Both groups of rats were injected with cancer cells. Roughly nine days after the cells were injected, 67% of the intermittent fasting rats survived, while only 21% of the ad libitum rats survived. At ten days post inoculation of the cancer cells, 50% of the intermittent fasting rats survived, and only 12.5% of the ad libitum rats survived. The authors concluded the following:

> *"Thus, the survival of tumor-bearing rats was enhanced by short-term relatively mild dietary restrictions. We suggest that relatively mild dietary restrictions should be included in clinical trials designed to inhibit cancer growth and enhance the survival of human cancer patients."*

Note that the authors refer to intermittent fasting as short-term mild dietary restriction, which is the same thing and shouldn't get confused. It is pretty cool how a dietary pattern performed for such a short period of time can have such major implications, like enhancing survival of cancer. I wonder if oncologists are aware of any of these studies?

Then there is this study out of the journal *Science Translational Medicine* where they show that not only can intermittent fasting protect normal cells from the harmful side effects of chemotherapy drugs, but fasting can also kill the cancer cells!

Remember that cancer cells lack the metabolic flexibility to use fat as fuel. They can only get their nutrition via sugar. This study expands on this concept, explaining how cancer cells lack the ability to respond and thrive under extreme environments. One of these extreme environments is starving the body of sugar, their primary energy source. Another one of these extreme environments is intermittent fasting.

Healthy cells have a normal feedback mechanism. When there is a lack of food, normal cells adapt and conserve resources and actually become stronger and healthier as a result. Cancer cells lack this feedback mechanism, as they prefer to feed continuously. Cancer cells are:

> *"Addicted to nutrients. When they can't consume enough, they begin to die. The addiction to nutrients explains why changes to metabolic pathways are so common and tend to arise first as a cell progresses toward cancer."*
> – Dr. Chi Van Dang, director of the Abramson Cancer Center at the University of Pennsylvania

The inability of cancer cells to respond properly to extreme environments does not allow them to adapt to the altered concentrations of sugar, growth factors, and other molecules caused by intermittent

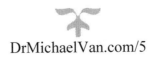

fasting. For example, tumor cells cannot adapt to the reduction of glucose, IGF-1, and other pro-growth proteins and factors that fasting causes. The cancerous cells respond to these changes through a series of cellular reactions resulting in an increase in oxidative stress, damage to their DNA, and eventually the cancer cells die.

This study also shows that intermittent fasting has the potential to enhance chemotherapy and can even take place of chemotherapy for early-stage cancer patients who do not require chemotherapy. In addition, this can be used for patients with advanced-stage cancer in combination with chemotherapy by slowing and possibly ceasing tumor progression, as well as reducing side effects of the drugs. In the authors' own words:

> *"These studies suggest that multiple cycles of fasting promote differential stress sensitization in a wide range of tumors and could potentially replace or augment the efficacy of certain chemotherapy drugs in the treatment of various cancers."*

You heard that right. Intermittent fasting has been shown to starve cancer cells while simultaneously protecting cells from chemotherapy toxicity! In fact, one research group is reportedly

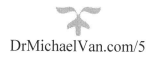

working on getting intermittent fasting approved by the US Food and Drug Administration (FDA) as an adjunct therapy for cancer patients.

The journal *Cell Metabolism* described three major factors that happen when initiating intermittent fasting for two cycles of four-day long fasts per month. First, this intermittent fasting regimen rejuvenates the immune system and reduces cancer incidence. Second, it causes beneficial changes in risk factors of age-related diseases in humans. Finally, it actually promotes neurogenesis of the hippocampus and improves cognitive performance in mice.

Remember when I discussed the brain function benefits of intermittent fasting in Chapter 5 and how the hippocampus is a special part of the brain that is located deep in the temporal lobes? It specifically deals with the formation of long-term memories and spatial navigation. Neurogenesis (the generation of new brain cells) in this area can lead to enhanced brain functioning in areas such as special learning, pattern discrimination, contextual memory and mood regulation.

Intermittent fasting literally produced multi-system regeneration in mice. Visceral belly fat, the harmful fat surrounding organs, was reduced, as well as the risk for cancer and inflammatory diseases declined. Meanwhile, immune and brain function improved, and

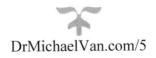

lifespan was increased. In the mouse brain, neurons were regenerated, improving learning, memory, and concentration. As if that wasn't enough, it also reduced the incidence of skin lesions and it ceased bone mineral density loss. It actually showed increases in healthy bone formation.

FIGURE 14.3: INTERMITTENT FASTING AND MULTI-SYSTEM REGENERATION

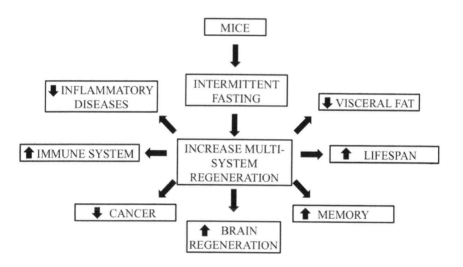

In part of this study discussing the pilot human trial, intermittent fasting decreased risk factors and biomarkers for aging, diabetes, cardiovascular disease, and cancer with no adverse side effects. The authors actually concluded that this provides support for the use of intermittent fasting not just to treat conditions like cancer, but to promote health period.

FIGURE 14.4: INTERMITTENT FASTING AND THE PROMOTION OF HEALTH

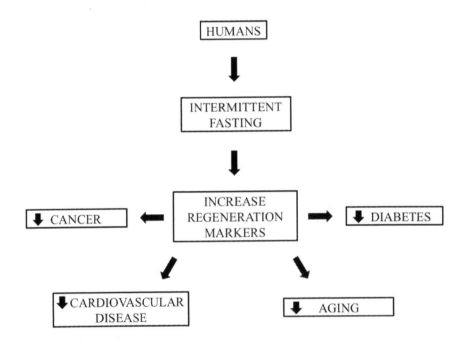

In the journal *Mechanisms of Ageing and Development*, they did a study that investigated the role of eating patterns on the prevention of age-related disorders. They showed that intermittent fasting for four months significantly reduced the incidence of lymphoma. Lymphoma is a group of blood cancers that develop in the lymphatic system. The two main types are Hodgkin lymphoma and non-Hodgkin lymphoma. Saying that fasting significantly reduced the incidence of lymphoma in this study doesn't do it justice. Not only did it reduce cancer, the intermittent fasting group actually had zero incidence of cancer, while the group eating freely had an incidence of 33%.

In addition, there was a huge decrease in the accumulation of free radicals, which is significant because high levels of free radicals are associated with aging. These results took place even though there was no difference in overall food consumption. The only difference was one group ate in a specific window, while the other group ate freely (ad libitum).

The study out of the journal *Teratogenesis Carcinogenesis and Mutagenesis* showed the same exact thing as the other studies and cannot be ignored. Intermittent fasting actually blocked the development of precancerous cells in the body, preventing cancer formation! This particular study focused on a specific cancer known as hepatocarcinogenesis, a fancy term for liver cancer. Their conclusion was that:

"Long-term IF regimen exerts an anti-promoting effect on rat hepatocarcinogenesis.."

You can say it with me… WOW!!! Who knew that all these studies existed in reputable peer-reviewed scientific journals? Who knew that something as simple as intermittent fasting could have such a profound effect on cancer? Think for a second if intermittent fasting combined with eliminating sugar was actually recommended to cancer patients. Can you imagine their results? They would absolutely put all these cancer drugs and chemotherapy to shame! This would actually result in the patient getting healthy instead of utilizing radiation and chemo which destroys the entire body and immune system. Not only that, utilizing intermittent fasting is free! Can you tell I'm excited? This needs to be public knowledge.

CHAPTER 15:

EPILEPSY

In the US, epilepsy affects an estimated 2.3 million adults and nearly 468,000 children below the age of 17. Epilepsy is a chronic neurological condition characterized by recurring seizures. It can have a significant impact on a person's quality of life, especially with the heightened risk of accidents and injuries these seizures can cause. Epilepsy can be very difficult to treat effectively. There are several types of seizures, and some children have multiple episodes every day. This disease is linked to periods of overexcitement in brain cells, causing uncontrolled jerking movements and loss of consciousness. It occurs most often in children.

There has been very promising research on the positive impact intermittent fasting can have on epilepsy patients. Numerous studies have shown how nerve cells in the brains of animals maintained on an intermittent fasting regimen exhibited increased resistance to neurotoxins relevant to epilepsy, Huntington's disease, Parkinson's disease, and Alzheimer's disease. This protection intermittent fasting has on brain cells is a large reason intermittent fasting can specifically help counteract these disease processes.

Healthy growth factors are believed to play a fundamental role in regulating a lot of these brain and nervous system disorders. This includes intermittent fasting's ability to increase the levels of BDNF (brain-derived neurotrophic factor) and GDNF (glial cell line-derived neurotrophic factor) in several regions of the brain. These growth factors serve to protect brain cells against various types of stress, including protection against conditions like epilepsy and other degenerative brain disorders. It has even been suggested that the increase in BDNF can actually enhance our body to become more insulin-sensitive. More on the mechanism of increased brain functioning from intermittent fasting is in the brain function section in Chapter 5.

KETOGENIC DIET & INTERMITTENT FASTING'S ROLE IN EPILEPSY

This is the main reason why ketogenic diet has also been associated with an improvement in the symptoms of epilepsy. Standard treatment for epilepsy includes anti-epileptic drugs, which is not effective in roughly 40% of patients. This type of epilepsy that is unresponsive to medication is called refractory epilepsy. When medication fails these patients, oftentimes, a ketogenic diet will take its place. A ketogenic diet calls for minimizing carbohydrates and replacing them with healthy fats and moderate amounts of high-quality protein. As we have already concluded, this diet will also help optimize your weight and virtually all chronic degenerative disease, as this type of diet will help you convert from burning carbs as your primary fuel to burning fat. Much more information on the ketogenic diet can be found in Chapters 6 and 14.

Traditionally, a ketogenic diet consists of a 3:1:1 or a 4:1:1 fat to carbohydrate and protein ratio, with 87-90 percent of total calories coming from fat. A modified Atkins diet has also been successfully used, which consists of a 1:1:1 fat to carb and protein ratio, with roughly 50 percent of total calories coming from fat.

Clinical medicine began recognizing the impact a ketogenic diet could have on the treatment of epilepsy in the late 90's. The American Epilepsy Society even has a Ketogenic Diet Special Interest Group organized by Dr. Thomas Seyfried, who today is one of the leading academic researchers looking at using the ketogenic diet as a cancer treatment. Another key player in this group was Jim Abrahams, who created the Charlie Foundation for his son Charlie, who went through a near-death experience from seizures. He was healed by implementing a ketogenic diet to control his seizures. Currently, a ketogenic diet is used as a first line approach in epilepsy when medications fail and is also very important in the management in seizures that are unresponsive to drugs.

In fact, one third of children who respond to the diet have a 90% or greater decrease in seizures. In one study, children treated with a ketogenic diet for three months had a 75% decrease in baseline seizures, on average. Although the classic ketogenic diet can be very effective against seizures, it requires close supervision by a neurologist and dietitian as the food choices are quite limited. The diet can be difficult to follow, particularly for older children and adults.

In many cases, the Modified Atkins diet (MAD) has proven to be as effective or nearly as effective for childhood seizure management as the classic ketogenic diet. The Modified Atkins diet also has fewer side effects and is a little less strict in nutrient ratios, adding to compliance. In an analysis of 10 studies comparing the classic ketogenic diet to the modified Atkins diet, people were much more likely to stick to the modified Atkins diet. In a randomized study of 102 children, 30% of those who followed the modified Atkins diet experienced a 90% or greater reduction in seizures.

Interestingly, the mechanism by which the ketogenic diet manages seizures is not nearly as clear as the way the ketogenic diet manages cancer. This is ironic considering that it's barely known, let alone applied, within the cancer industry, while it's already an established treatment for epilepsy.

A ketogenic diet has a successful track record of treating epileptic children, but adult studies have also recently come to light, even though they are more limited. According to a recent review of the published studies, the authors explained how adults who followed a ketogenic diet typically experienced rapid and beneficial results. According to the authors:

> *"The anticonvulsant effect occurs quickly with both diets, within days to weeks. Side effects of both diets are benign and similar. The most serious, hyperlipidemia, reverses with treatment*

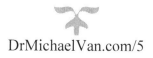

discontinuation. The most common, weight loss, may be
advantageous in patients with obesity...

In summary, ketogenic and modified Atkins diet treatment show
modest efficacy, although in some patients the effect is
remarkable. The diets are well-tolerated, but often discontinued
because of their restrictiveness. In patients willing to try dietary
treatment, the effect is seen quickly, giving patients the option
whether to continue the treatment."

What was also interesting about the findings is that many
children remain seizure free after discontinuing the diet, but not so much
with adults. Adult epileptics likely need to maintain the diet indefinitely
in order to not suffer a relapse in seizures.

Most people out there are adapted to burning carbohydrates as
their primary fuel instead of burning fat. This is a result of eating a diet
too high in sugar and carbs and lacking healthy fats. This is devastating
to one's health, as the most common side effect is insulin and leptin
resistance, which is at the root of all chronic disease.

One of the best strategies to speed up your body's ability to burn
fat as your primary fuel over carbohydrates is to combine a ketogenic
diet with intermittent fasting. This will up-regulate the enzymes that are

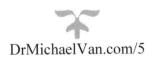

used to burn fat as fuel, and down-regulate your glucose enzymes. Intermittent fasting can help you make a gradual transition to a ketogenic diet because it breaks your body's addiction to glucose. In fact, removing your cravings for sugar is one of the most common benefits of intermittent fasting.

Keep in mind here that while performing intermittent fasting with a ketogenic diet, two factors are important: what you eat, and when you eat. I have seen some people recommend eating all kinds of junk food while intermittent fasting, but I view this as counterproductive. You are what you eat at the end of the day. Although studies have shown decent results from eating "junk" while intermittent fasting, this will not allow you to become healthy in the process.

A ketogenic diet is actually very similar to what is ideal for human health. Combined with intermittent fasting, the results and benefits will be numerous. The primary difference here between someone who has a chronic disease such as epilepsy or cancer and people who have no such disease is how strict this regimen is maintained. Obviously, if you have a chronic disease such as epilepsy, you would want to maintain this as long as it takes to resolve insulin resistance. However, this regimen is good for anyone trying to get healthy and stay healthy, it just doesn't need to be super consistent and can be open to allow occasional cheat days. You also can be more lenient on the specific nutrient ratios for the maintenance health, including allowing more protein and healthy carbohydrates from fruits and vegetables in your diet.

CHAPTER 16:

INTERMITTENT FASTING PLANS

When you begin to start implementing intermittent fasting into your lifestyle, consider the following methods on the next few pages:

1. DAILY INTERMITTENT FASTING

This is the most common plan that I personally recommend. This is the plan of fasting that I abide by and further discuss in Chapter 18 where I talk specifically about my personal plan. I find it to be the most natural way to implement fasting and find it is very effortless.

The most common approach to incorporate daily intermittent fasting is to restrict daily eating to a specific window of time. To be effective, the length of your daily fast must be at least 16 hours for men and around 14 hours for women. Generally, women seem to get better results when they implement slightly shorter fasting periods. Therefore, your daily eating window would be a maximum of 8 hours for males and 10 hours for females.

Within the eating window, you can fit two or three meals in, depending on what works best for you. This method of fasting can actually be as easy as skipping breakfast. For those who get hungry in the morning and like to eat breakfast, this can be a little hard to get used to at first. However, after a few weeks, the hunger cravings usually subside.

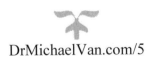

This is the plan I refer to a lot throughout this book because it is the most widely accepted strategy by many experts. I personally recommend skipping breakfast, although you can theoretically skip dinner as well. Here is an example of the most common fasting protocol where you skip breakfast or dinner:

- **Skipping Breakfast Fast**

    12-1 PM:
    - First Meal (largest meal of the day)

    4 PM:
    - Second meal (optional)

    7-8 PM:
    - Last meal before the fast

    8 PM-12 PM Next Day:
    - 16 hour fasting period

- **Skipping Dinner Fast**

    7-8 AM:

    o   First Meal (largest meal of the day)

    11 AM:

    o   Second meal (optional)

    2-3 PM:

    o   Last meal before the fast

    3 PM-7 AM Next Day:

    o   16 hour fasting period

These are all examples and you don't necessarily have to follow just one all the time. You have the freedom here to switch it up, although I would recommend picking one and sticking with it.

As we have discussed, there are a ton of benefits if you exercise in a fasted state. Benefits include but are not limited to increasing your natural production of human growth hormone and increasing the amount of fat you burn. Following are some examples of different protocols you can model if you add in an exercise program, which are similar to the leangains protocol developed by fitness expert Martin Berkhan:

- **Fasted Training**

    11:30 AM:
    - o 10 g BCAA (optional)

    12-1 PM:
    - o Training

    1 PM:
    - o Post-workout meal (largest meal of the day)

    4 PM:
    - o Second meal (optional)

    8-9 PM:
    - o Last meal before the fast

    9 PM-1 PM Next Day:
    - o 16 hour fasting period

- **Early Morning Fasted Training**

  5:30 AM:

  - 10 g BCAA (optional)

  6-7 AM:

  - Training

  8 AM:

  - 10 g BCAA (optional)

  10 AM:

  - 10 g BCAA (optional)

  12-1 PM:

  - The main post-workout meal (largest meal of the day). The beginning of the 8 hour eating window

  7-8 PM:

  - Last meal before the fast

  8 PM-12 PM Next Day:

  - 16 hour fasting period

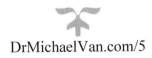

- **One Pre-Workout Meal**

  12-1 PM:

  - o Pre-workout meal. Approximately 20-25% of daily total calorie intake.

  3-4 PM:

  - o Training should happen a few hours after the pre-workout meal.

  4-5 PM:

  - o Post-workout meal (largest meal).

  7-8 PM:

  - o Last meal before the fast.

  8 PM-12 PM Next Day:

  - o 16 Hour Fasted Period

- **Two Pre-Workout Meals**

12-1 PM:

  o Meal number one. Approximately 20-25% of daily total calorie intake.

3-4 PM:

  o Pre-workout meal. Roughly equal to the first meal.

6-7 PM:

  o Training

7-8 PM:

  o Post-workout meal (largest meal)

8 PM-12 PM Next Day:

  o 16 Hour Fasted Period

It is important to note that the last two examples involving pre-workout meals are less effective and not recommended. I believe (and scientific research backs this) that a pre-workout meal can be counterproductive to increasing growth hormone and negate a lot of fat loss benefits. Training in a fasted state is simply the best way to get the best physiological benefits for your body, so that is what I stick to. As you can see, you can choose to go about your fast in a variety of different ways. Since daily exercise is a genetic requirement for expressing optimal health, I organize my fasting regimen around my exercise, period.

BCAA's in the above protocols stand for branched chain amino acids. These are generally used for protein intake to stimulate protein synthesis and metabolism during your fasted state before a workout. It also helps with increased phosphorylation, which is an indicator of muscle growth. BCAA's allow faster transport of amino acids, the building blocks of protein, into muscle cell membranes.

When I talk about incorporating BCAA's, I am assuming that you have the desired outcome of getting as lean and strong as possible. It is highly recommended to take BCAA's around

30 minutes before your workout. Note: they are not counted towards your fasting period. In addition, if you are unable to consume a meal after a workout (like in the early morning fasted training example above), then I would take BCAA's after as well to keep stimulating muscle and protein synthesis and avoiding muscle wasting.

If you are just looking for a specific eating regimen without the training aspect, that is fine. My recommendation is to stay firm to the eight hour feeding window and you can always incorporate the fasted training aspect later if desired.

With that said, you can also restrict your eating window even further to get better results, such as going down to six, four, or even two hours. However, the fact that you can still reap many of these benefits by just utilizing the eight hour protocol is why it is the most popular. As an example, you only eat between the hours of 11am until 7pm. This boils down to skipping breakfast and making lunch your first meal of the day. This specific plan is promoted in the book, "The 8-Hour Diet," by David Zinczenko and Peter Moore. It is also promoted by Martin Berkhan's leangains protocol and Dr. Mercola.

It doesn't matter when you start your 8-hour eating period. If you desire, you can start at 8am and stop at 4pm. Or you can start at 2pm and stop at 10pm. Do whatever works for you and is easiest to implement into your schedule. For myself, breakfast is the easiest meal to skip.

Doing intermittent fasting everyday makes it easy to become a daily habit. It is one less thing to think about when incorporating this new aspect of your healthy lifestyle. You probably already eat around the same time every day without even thinking about it. It is the exact same thing here with daily intermittent fasting. You will just become accustomed to not eating at certain times.

One potential disadvantage of this type of schedule is for those who maybe don't want to lose any weight or fat. This may apply to an elite athlete, or someone who is completely satisfied with their body composition and current fitness level. These people may still choose to implement intermittent fasting for the other numerous benefits, such as enhanced growth hormone production or boosting brain function, but just not this specific plan of doing it everyday. For these people, cutting out a meal everyday may make it more difficult to consume the same number of calories as before. It may be a little challenging to teach yourself to consume larger meals on a consistent basis to make up for the one missed. Therefore, this plan can really be a good thing or potentially a bad thing, depending on your goals.

2. THE 5:2 PLAN

The following is an excerpt taken from a study out of the *British Journal of Diabetes & Vascular Disease*:

> *"Intermittent fasting can be undertaken in several ways but the basic format alternates days of 'normal' calorie consumption with days when calorie consumption is severely restricted. This can either be done on an alternating day basis, or more recently a 5:2 strategy has been developed [see figure below], where 2 days each week are classed as 'fasting days' (with <600 calories consumed for men, <500 for women). Importantly,* **this type of intermittent fasting has been shown to be similarly effective or more effective than continuous modest calorie restriction** *with regard to weight loss, improved insulin sensitivity and other health biomarkers... Despite the seemingly strict nature of the fasting days intermittent fasting has a generally good adherence record."*

This specific intermittent fasting schedule was popularized by Dr. Michael Mosley in his diet book, "The Fast

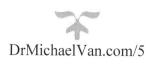

Diet: Lose Weight, Stay Healthy, and Live Longer with the Simple Secret of Intermittent Fasting." Dr. Mosley, one of the study's researchers, claims to have lost 19 pounds in two months by following this recommendation. In this plan, you are allowed to eat normally five days a week and you only fast on two. On the fasting days, you restrict your calories down to ¼ of your normal food intake. This equates to about 600 calories in men and 500 for women, along with plenty of water and tea.

For example, you may choose to fast on Mondays and Thursdays, where you eat two small meals that are around 250 calories per meal for women and 300 calories per meal for men. This would mean that the other five days you would just eat a normal diet. Personally, I hate using the word "normal" when describing the concept of eating around the clock. It may be the common form of eating in today's society, but it doesn't mean it's normal. This is especially true when you look at our ancestor's dieting pattern who did not have access to food every hour of the day.

This type of plan has been shown to have similar benefits (and superior benefits in some cases) as continuous calorie restriction, including improvements in weight loss, insulin

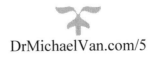

sensitivity, and other biomarkers for health. With that said, it becomes challenging to make it a habit for most people, as it is not implemented daily.

For those who tend to go out, splurge, and enjoy their weekends, choosing the two fasting days on the weekdays may be a good idea. With this plan, it may increase compliance doing the fasting days on the weekdays and leaving the weekends open for normal eating and activity. It will simply be less of a shock to the system to get the ball rolling.

3. ALTERNATE DAY INTERMITTENT FASTING

This is the least common method where you alternate fasting days every other day. You can either treat this as the daily intermittent fasting method or the 5:2 fasting method. What I mean by that is you can treat the fasting days as days where you eat during a specific time window outlined in the daily fasting method (#1) or you can treat the fast consuming only 500-600 calories based on the 5:2 plan (#2).

For example, you can eat normally on Monday, fast on Tuesday, and continue that pattern for the rest of the week. On your fasting days, you can either choose to narrow your eating window to roughly 8 hours like in the first plan outlined, or you can limit your calories to 500-600 mentioned in the second plan outlined.

This can also involve a 24-hour fast followed by a 24-hour non-fasting period. This is sometimes referred to as every other day fasting or every other day feeding. A full fast every other day is rather extreme for my liking, and do not recommend this, especially for beginners. You will end up going to bed very hungry several times a week, which is not pleasant at all and most likely will be unsustainable in the long-term.

Similar to the 5:2 plan, this type of fasting regimen doesn't allow a habitual pattern of consistency, so it is hard to incorporate it into your lifestyle for long periods of time. For me personally, this plan is much too sporadic.

4. EAT-STOP-EAT FASTING

This type of fasting regimen, popularized by fitness expert Brad Pilon, involves fasting for 24 hours, once or twice a week. It is similar to the 5:2 plan, but you consume absolutely no calories during the fasted days (vs 500-600 calories in the 5:2 plan). For example, you would not eat from dinner one day until dinner the following day, amounting to a 24-hour fast. Let's say you want to start your first day of fasting and finish dinner on Monday around 7pm. Then you wouldn't eat again until Tuesday at 7pm. You can also fast from breakfast to breakfast, or lunch to lunch. The end result will still be the same.

If you are doing this for weight loss, it is important to eat "normally" during the eating periods. In other words, try not to overeat during your 24-hour eating periods. The problem with this method is that a full 24-hour fast is very difficult for most people. You can always start with a 14-16 hour fast and then move upwards from there if a full 24 hours is too hard. Personally, I find that this is easy to do during the first 16-18 hours, but the last few hours are very difficult and I get extremely fatigued, grouchy, and hungry. It does indeed take a lot of self-discipline to finish the full 24-hour fast.

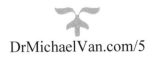

5. THE WARRIOR DIET

"Our ancestors consumed food much less frequently and often had to subsist on one large meal per day, and thus from an evolutionary perspective, human beings were adapted to intermittent feeding rather than to grazing."
- (Mattson, M.P., PhD, Lancet 2005)

The Warrior Diet was popularized by fitness expert Ori Hofmekler. It involves eating small amounts of raw fruits and vegetables during the daytime, then eating one huge meal at night. Technically you are not fasting to the full extent here, because you do allow very small amounts of fruit and vegetables. The diet calls for minimizing your food intake to small servings of fresh fruits, vegetables and light fast assimilating protein such as whey protein, yogurt or kefir in the morning and afternoon. Avoid grains, meats and refined food during as well as sugary treats and beverages during this time period.

You feast at night within a four hour eating window. This is the time for your main meal where you're allowed to eat as much as you desire as long as you keep the right food

combinations. You stop eating when you feel pleasantly
satisfied or when you get substantially more thirsty than hungry.

The diet emphasizes food choices that are quite similar to
a paleo diet. This diet is based on the types of foods presumed to
have been eaten by Paleolithic humans that works most with our
genetics. It consists of whole, unprocessed foods, healthy meat,
fish, vegetables, and fruit. It doesn't involve dairy or grain
products. It is high in fat, moderate in animal protein, and low to
moderate in carbohydrates.

6. SPONTANEOUS MEAL SKIPPING

This plan does not involve any structured intermittent fasting regimen in order to gain some of the benefits. Notice I say "some" of the benefits. It won't give you the results of applying the daily intermittent fasting plan, but it can be a good start. It basically translates into a "skip meals when convenient" plan. If you are not hungry one day, skip breakfast and just consume a healthy lunch and dinner. If you are busy travelling and don't have time to eat, do a short fast.

When you end up skipping a meal or two, you are essentially doing a spontaneous intermittent fast. Just make sure you eat healthy foods at the other meals.

CHAPTER 17:

IMPLEMENTATION

Why do intermittent fasting? Besides the numerous benefits listed previously, it drastically simplifies your day. Instead of having to prepare, time, and eat meals every 2-3 hours, you only have to focus on eating during your short eating window. It requires a lot less time in preparation because instead of dropping what you are doing to eat 6 times a day, you only have to do this 2 or 3 times. Instead of doing the dishes 6 times a day, you only have to do it 2 or 3 times.

Probably the biggest concern out there is that this type of eating plan will cause your energy and focus to go down the drain and cause a huge spike in your hunger. You might be thinking, "even when I skip breakfast once, my hunger spikes drastically and my stomach starts to grumble. How on Earth do you expect me to do this all the time? I'm going to feel miserable every morning, and therefore, I am going to feel miserable at work and my productivity will take a big hit." Relax and stay calm.

You can drink water, coffee, and other non-caloric beverages during the fast. This can help reduce hunger cravings. During your eating window, focus on healthy foods for best results. This simply won't work as well if you eat tons of junk food or excessive amounts of calories.

Indeed, as with any new major lifestyle change, you will have to fight through an initial transition period. Going from an eating all-the-time regimen to intermittent fasting can be a big jolt to the system. The grouchy and hungry feeling you get when you skip a meal initially is a direct response to your eating habits. Your body in this stage is expecting food every 2-3 hours because that is what you have always done. If you have eaten breakfast every day of your life, your body will be expecting breakfast when you wake up. However, once you get through that initial transition period, your body will actually learn to function better. Remember when discussing the fat burning benefit, it takes an average of two weeks to give your body enough time to learn how to effectively burn fat as fuel instead of carbohydrate (blood sugar and muscle glycogen).

According to research published in 2010, if you practice intermittent fasting followed by periods of overeating, the benefits go down the drain. This seems like an obvious statement, but it is an important one. When you gorge excessively during your non-fasting days or non-fasting hours, the health benefits can easily be lost. You can gain benefits if you consume the same or less calories than the amount of calories you ate before. You just can't consume more calories and expect to get amazing results.

During the initial two week transition, one typically does have sugar and hunger cravings, as well as experiencing a dip in energy levels. To counteract these feelings, you can use coconut oil or grass-fed butter as a healthy short and medium-chain fat to relieve these cravings and dip in energy you may experience. This type of healthy fat is rapidly broken down in the body and can supply your body with some much-needed fuel. It will also provide you with a source of energy until your body can effectively burn your own fat.

What I personally do is consume organic black coffee in the morning blended together with healthy fats. The personal recipe I use for my coffee calls for organic black coffee blended with one tablespoon of grass-fed raw butter and one tablespoon of coconut oil. I will also add a pinch of cinnamon for more flavor. There is absolutely no protein or carbohydrates in this coffee, so it will not allow your insulin levels to spike. If your insulin levels do not spike, you will continue to burn fat as your primary fuel. This allows your body to stay in a fasted state, reaping all the benefits outlined in this book.

Grass-fed high-quality butter (preferably not pasteurized) not only has a massive impact on cognitive function, but it gives you many of the benefits of raw healthy milk fat without the damaging denatured casein proteins. This type of butter can usually be found at a local farmers market. If you can't find it there, then you can opt for Kerry Gold grass-fed Irish butter found in almost every local grocery store. It is pasteurized, but it is far superior in my opinion to anything else you can get. Grass-fed butter contains omega-3 fatty acids, CLA (conjugated linolenic acid), beta-carotene, vitamin A, vitamin K2, vitamin D, vitamin E, and antioxidants. It is high in a special short-chain fatty acid known as butyrate, or butyric acid. This improves body composition, increases metabolism, improves gut health, and protects the functioning of your brain.

The coconut oil gives you a rich source of medium chain triglycerides. Healthy medium-chained fats are easily converted into energy at a much faster rate than longer chain fats. Within minutes of consuming coconut oil, your body is able to process these fats and spike

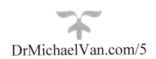

up your ketone levels, the preferred energy source for the majority of your heart and brain. This means that you will halt the feeling of low energy and increased hunger. It will reset your hormone levels so you can stay in a high-energy fat-burning mode without that undesired light-headed and hungry feeling.

When you have decided you are ready to give intermittent fasting a try, consider taking the first step of skipping breakfast. The fasting period at night and the first thing in the morning is a great opportunity to be productive and get things done. Try and keep busy instead of sitting around in boredom sulking about food.

The largest amount of calories consumed during the day will be the first meal at lunch time, ideally after your exercise period. Refer to the sample protocols on intermittent fasting in Chapter 15. Even if you are taking a rest day from exercise, try and make the first meal of the day your largest meal. A general rule of thumb is to consume at least 35-40% of your daily calories during your first meal of the day. If this is too hard to do, then don't worry. You can still have your largest meal in the evening instead of 12PM. Some people prefer their largest meal of the day being at dinner time on rest days with their family instead of a large lunch. If that makes you consistent with the diet and abide by the eight hour window of eating, then that is completely fine.

Make sure you restrict your eating to an 8-hour time frame every day. In the 6-8 hour eating window, consume moderate amounts of healthy protein, minimize carbohydrates like pasta, potatoes, and bread, and consume an abundance of healthy fats. Healthy fats can include grass-fed raw butter, eggs, avocados, coconut oil, olive oil, nuts, and seeds. Other oils can include grape seed oil, avocado oil, and macadamia nut oil. What this comes down to is loading up on most of your calories in the form of healthy fats, the exact same fats that the media and the so-called "experts" tell you to avoid in your diet. This will further shift your body from carb burning to an efficient fat burning machine.

In addition to intermittent fasting, I believe you can eliminate almost all sickness and disease and improve your health by taking the following into account:

- Carbohydrates and Sugar
  - Consume in the form of lots of vegetables and fruits. Reduce and even consider eliminating processed foods, sugar/fructose, and grain based foods. Even unprocessed organic grains spike up your insulin levels pushing you into the stress response. Cancer cells only get their nutrition via fructose, so if you want to avoid cancer, you

need to avoid all forms of sugar. Aim for a total fructose level of around 25 grams a day.

- Fat
    - Replace excessive carbohydrates and protein with healthy fats, such as organic eggs from pastured hens, avocados, coconut oil, nuts and seeds, grass-fed butter, and high-quality meats. Also optimize your omega-3 to omega-6 ratio by consuming high quality krill oil and wild salmon, while reducing your intake of processed vegetable oils.

- Probiotics
    - Enhancing your gut bacteria will not only reduce unhealthy inflammation levels of the body, but also strengthen your immune response. Many harmful bacteria that get colonized into the gut from an unhealthy lifestyle actually can cause a chronic inflammatory response and fuel the development and growth of cancer cells. Following the guidelines under "MICROBIOME CHANGES" in Chapter 6 will actually slow cancer progression and can improve the response to chemotherapy.

- Exercise
    - Exercise was found to not only enhance your healthy gut bacteria, but it also lowers insulin levels. Insulin and a high sugar environment encourages growth and spread of cancer. Exercise also enhances immune cells, making them more potent with the capability to fight diseases like cancer. Exercise can actually help trigger cell death of cancer cells, a process called apoptosis. Shoot for a well-rounded exercise program that includes balance, strength, flexibility, and high intensity interval training (HIIT). This will be covered in more detail in my next book.

- Sunshine
    - There is massive evidence out there that shows how vitamin D can decrease your risk of cancer by more than half. Ideally, you want your blood level of vitamin D to be at 50-70 ng/ml. If you are being treated for cancer, than it might be more advantageous to have a level of 80-90 ng/ml. If you live in an area without optimal sun exposure (where your shadow is longer than your body height) or when it is winter, it is necessary to supplement with vitamin D. When supplementing with vitamin D,

make sure to combine it with Vitamin K2 in the form of MK-7, as these vitamins work synergistically in the body.

- Sleep
    - Poor sleep has many negative health effects on the body, including messing up your body's ability to make melatonin (sleep hormone). It also increases your risk of having insulin resistance and weight gain, which we already know raises the risk of cancer.

What to avoid:

- Processed Foods
    - Processed foods such as excessive amounts of grains and sugars feed your pathogenic bacteria.

- Antibacterial Soaps
    - These soaps kill off both your bad and good bacteria, and overtime can contribute to antibiotic resistance.

- GMOs
    - Avoid genetically modified foods at all costs, as they are treated with glyphosate (Roundup), which is a

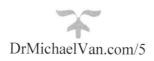

carcinogen. Replace with fresh, organic, locally grown foods.

- Toxins
  - Limiting exposure to toxins is crucial. These include pesticides, herbicides, household chemical cleaners, toxic cosmetics, many plastics, and synthetic air fresheners.

- Chlorinated And / Or Fluoridated Water
  - Chlorine / fluoride kills not only the pathogenic bacteria in water but it also kills the beneficial bacteria in your gut. Look for quality water filtration systems or get your water at a local water store.

- Antibiotics
  - There are exceptions to every rule, but generally you want to avoid these unless absolutely necessary. If you do choose to use them, it is important to make sure you take it with fermented foods and / or a probiotic supplement to help replenish your gut.

- Conventionally Raised Meats
  - This includes all animal products from concentrated animal feeding operations (CAFO). It is routine at these feeding lots to feed low-dose antibiotics to these animals that aid in the destruction of your gut. Coupled with genetically engineered grains that the animals consume, this makes CAFO animals very dangerous.

CHAPTER 18:

MY PERSONAL PLAN

I am a firm believer of daily productive habits, especially habits that involve my body and health. As a Christian, I love the verses of 1 Corinthians 6:19-20. It reads, "Don't you realize that your body is the temple of the Holy Spirit, who lives in you and was given to you by God? …. So you must honor God with your body." I was given this body of mine as a gift from God, so I am going to honor that body by taking care of it to the best of my ability and making it as healthy as possible. That is why I choose to take daily measures of healthy living. Not twice a week like the 5:2 plan. Not every other day, but every day. With all the healthy benefits intermittent fasting has to offer, I choose to incorporate it every day to give my body the most optimal health benefits.

Since intermittent fasting is more of a lifestyle change than a diet, you need to make it a habit. I believe that doing a regimen where you fast one day, take the next day off, and fast the following day is not sustainable. You will never make this a habit if you choose this method, which is why I recommend against it. When you do the same thing every day, it takes the thought process out of the equation because we move into autopilot. It allows us to form a habit.

I keep my eight hour feeding window constant to the protocol I outline below due to the hormonal pattern of meal frequency. For example, ghrelin, the hormone in your body that induces hunger, starts to adapt its release to your daily eating habits. When I have a pattern of always consuming my first and largest meal around 12 PM, the physiology of my body adapts to this frequency by preparing for the meal and releasing these hunger hormones at that time. Eventually on this plan we will get hungry the same time everyday, simplifying things. If we eat sporadically throughout the day, ghrelin release cannot be controlled because there has been no orderly pattern to adjust to.

Patients ask me all the time, "when is the best time of day to workout?" I tell them it doesn't matter, as long as they try and do it the same time each day. That way it gets engrained into their subconscious and it becomes extremely easy to implement.

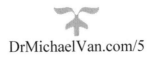

The intermittent fasting plan I choose to abide by is the daily 16 hour fast. I eat the same number of calories as I used to before, but instead of eating all day long, I condense all my calorie consumption into an eight hour window. This is what my schedule looks like on the following page:

- 4-5:00 AM:
  - Wake up
- 11:00 AM:
  - Pre-workout drink consisting of 7-10 g BCAA
- 11:30 AM:
  - Work out utilizing specific techniques to focus on muscle building and strength by optimizing human growth hormone release.
  - This type of workout is known as high intensity interval training (HIIT Training) and I will discuss this method in detail in my next publication.
- 12:00 PM:
  - Immediately consume about half of my calories for the day.
  - I first consume a massive calorie-dense post-workout smoothie with grass-fed whey protein concentrate, coconut oil, and superfoods.
  - This is followed by a whole-food meal
- 7:00 PM
  - Consume the second half of my calories for the day in the form of a large whole-food dinner
- 7:30 / 8:00 PM – 12:00 PM the next day
  - Fasting period of 16 hours

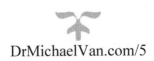

DrMichaelVan.com/5

This way works best for me because I would rather start my fast earlier in my day rather than later. This is mostly because of behavioral and social reasons. I prefer to have a nice dinner at night with my wife, then go to bed around 9:00 PM satiated. It is also easier for me to skip breakfast because my day starts off at such a busy pace that I don't have time to think about food during my grind-it-out schedule. Later in the evening is my time to unwind and consume a nice large meal.

This lifestyle change that I have incorporated daily for the last three years has changed my life. Initially, I was able to put on a very large amount of lean muscle mass. It changed my whole thought process and philosophy on muscle building and fat loss. As a former athletic trainer, this went against everything I thought was correct. To this day, I am able to easily maintain and still gain minor improvements as I continue with daily intermittent fasting. I continue to build lean muscle mass and lose fat mass at the same time.

My personal goals are to continue to build lean body mass as well as maintain the results I already have. Research has shown that fasted training positively influences your post-workout muscle building response in comparison to training while in a fed state. Fasted training makes the post-workout meal absolutely crucial, as this meal will directly influence the stimulation of protein synthesis in your muscle.

INTERMITTENT FASTING VS BULK AND CUT METHOD

While I'm at it discussing my personal regimen, I have to explain the traditional method of getting "cut and shredded." Many people follow the bulk up and cut technique. This is where you start in a phase of weight gain where you overeat and gain as much mass as possible in the form muscle and a lot of fat. After you reach the amount of muscle mass you desire, you then go into the cutting phase where you cut calories to lose fat, and consequently, some muscle mass as well. The end result after this method is settling at a higher weight than you were initially with more muscle.

Now, this method can work, and has worked for some people, especially athletes in physique competitions. However, the swing in weight is crazy. It's not uncommon to see people put on 25 lbs in the bulking phase and then in the cutting phase losing 20 lbs. The net result of this major swing in body weight is a muscle gain of 5 lbs. In the mean time, your body is going through crazy swings in body mass, causing your clothes to fit differently. Your body is constantly changing its level of composition, and throughout this process your body will wonder what the heck is going on with all these major swings.

Intermittent fasting is superior because you avoid this massive swing in weight because you can easily maintain the muscle building and fat loss results at the same time. You also end up eating more and spending more on food than you would by training with intermittent fasting. Instead of overeating to gain two pounds of muscle and six pounds of fat in a month or so, you only eat just enough to put on two pounds of muscle without adding any fat. Yes, in order to gain muscle you do need to know what you are doing and implement specific strategies. If you are going for the extreme fitness results that I personally strive for, you can do this with intermittent fasting. It's a consistent, slow, and steady building process without major fluctuations in body composition.

Finally, what is nice about intermittent fasting compared to the bulk and cut method is there is never a need to get "vacation-ready" or get that summer body you have always dreamed for. Everyone wants to look good with a shirt off or in a bathing suit. With intermittent fasting where you can add muscle without adding the fat, you don't have to worry about this. The difference with the bulk and cut approach is you don't have to drastically alter your diet and go through time-consuming crazy extremes of major weight gain followed by significant periods of weight loss. By utilizing intermittent fasting and exercise, you keep your body fat percentage to a minimum, build strength and muscle, and if there is a little extra fat you notice around the mid-section, you just fine tune the diet a little bit to get the desired result. Then within a couple weeks, you should be back to the preferred body fat percentage you desire.

CHAPTER 19:

SAFETY AND SIDE EFFECTS

Intermittent fasting may not be for everyone. In fact, some people should be careful with intermittent fasting or avoid it altogether. For example, if you are underweight, or have had a history of eating problems and disorders, then you should not do intermittent fasting without first consulting with a health professional. In this type of case, intermittent fasting can actually do more harm than good.

It has been mentioned, on rare occasions, that it may not be quite as beneficial for women to fast. Albeit rare, it was shown in a rat trial to actually worsen blood sugar control. In addition, there have been a few instances where intermittent fasting can make female rats abnormally thin, weak, masculinized, infertile and cause them to miss cycles.

Although there are no human studies showing this, it is still important to be aware of this possibility.

Some anecdotal reports from women say they became amenorrheic (their menstrual period stopped) when they first started intermittent fasting, but then it went back to normal once they stopped doing it. Therefore, women should be a little more mindful to their body's reaction when intermittent fasting. My suggestion is that women ease into it, starting with longer eating windows in the range of 10-12 hours and slowly working your way down.

If you are trying to conceive, then consider halting intermittent fasting temporarily. Intermittent fasting is not recommended when pregnant or breastfeeding as it is most important to make sure you have enough proper nutrition to feed yourself and the baby.

While there are numerous benefits to intermittent fasting, I do not recommend this lifestyle for anyone who is underweight or has a history of eating disorders. On the contrary, please seek help from a medical professional to maximize your mental and physical state.

As I stated before, the main side effect of intermittent fasting is hunger. You may feel weak and light headed, but realize that this is

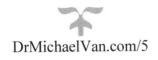

only be temporary. Once you allow your body time to adapt to using fat as its primary fuel, you will actually feel better than you did before.

If you have a medical condition, then you should consult with your doctor before trying intermittent fasting. This can include:

- Diabetes
- Blood sugar problems
- Low blood pressure
- Taking medications
- Underweight
- History of eating disorders
- Female and trying to conceive
- Female with a history of amenorrhea
- Pregnant or breastfeeding.

With all that said, intermittent fasting has an outstanding safety profile. If you are a healthy and well-nourished individual, there is nothing dangerous about not eating for a relatively short period of time.

CHAPTER 20:

COMMON QUESTIONS

1. Can I drink liquids during the fast?

    - Yes. Water, coffee, tea, and other non-caloric beverages
      are fine. Do not add any sugar to your coffee. A small
      amount of coconut oil, grass-fed butter, or cream may be
      okay. Coffee with healthy fats can actually be very
      beneficial during a fast because it can actually help give
      you energy and reduce your hunger.

2. Is it unhealthy to skip breakfast?

- No. The problem is that most people you hear of skipping breakfast have very unhealthy lifestyles. If you consume a healthy diet, you have nothing to worry about. Remember, breakfast foods became so popular based on ads paid for by the breakfast food companies themselves. It wasn't based on scientific evidence.

3. Can I take supplements while fasting?

- Yes. Just keep in mind that some supplements, especially fat-soluble vitamins, work and absorb a lot better when taken with meals. Therefore, most of my vitamins and supplements are taken during my first meal of the day to increase bioavailability.

4. Can I work out while fasted?

- Yes, fasted workouts are fine. In fact, they are encouraged for best results. I personally recommend taking branched-chain amino acids (BCAA's) before a fasted workout to ensure maximum muscle retention.

5. Will fasting cause muscle loss?

- All weight loss methods can theoretically cause muscle loss. With that said, studies have shown that intermittent fasting holds on to more than 50% more muscle mass than other conventional weight loss programs. Performing resistance training while intermittent fasting will allow you to hold on to even more muscle mass. Also, make sure you consume high-quality protein as part of your diet, especially after a workout. This will have a muscle-sparing effect on the body.

6. Will fasting slow down my metabolism?

- No. In fact, studies show that intermittent fasting actually boosts metabolism. With that said, fasts lasting longer than three days actually result in a suppressed metabolism, so it is best that you stick to one of the programs that I have outlined in this book. Remember, eating many small meals throughout the day to keep your metabolism up is a complete myth.

7. Should kids fast?

- No. Consuming a healthy diet to ensure proper growth and nutrition is the most important thing to do at that age group.

REFERENCES:

1.   Aksungar, F. B., Eren, A., Ure, S., Teskin, O., & Ates, G. (2005). Effects of
Intermittent Fasting on Serum Lipid Levels, Coagulation Status and Plasma
Homocysteine Levels. Annals of Nutrition and Metabolism Ann Nutr Metab,
49(2), 77-82. doi:10.1159/00008473

2.   Aksungar, F. B., Topkaya, A. E., & Akyildiz, M. (2007). Interleukin-6, C-
Reactive Protein and Biochemical Parameters during Prolonged Intermittent
Fasting. Annals of Nutrition and Metabolism Ann Nutr Metab, 51(1), 88-95.
doi:10.1159/000100954

3.   Alirezaei, M., Kemball, C. C., Flynn, C. T., Wood, M. R., Whitton, J. L., &
Kiosses, W. B. (2010). Short-term fasting induces profound neuronal autophagy.
Autophagy, 6(6), 702-710. doi:10.4161/auto.6.6.12376

4.   Antoni, R., Johnston, K., Collins, A., & Robertson, M. D. (2014). The Effects of
Intermittent Energy Restriction on Indices of Cardiometabolic Health. ENDO
Research in Endocrinology, 1-24. doi:10.5171/2014.459119

5.   Azevedo, F. R., Ikeoka, D., & Caramelli, B. (2013). Effects of intermittent
fasting on metabolism in men. Revista Da Associação Médica Brasileira
(English Edition), 59(2), 167-173. doi:10.1016/s2255-4823(13)70451-x

6.   Barnosky, A. R., Hoddy, K. K., Unterman, T. G., & Varady, K. A. (2014).
Intermittent fasting vs daily calorie restriction for type 2 diabetes prevention: A
review of human findings. Translational Research, 164(4), 302-311.
doi:10.1016/j.trsl.2014.05.013

7.   Baum, J.I., Layman, D.K., Freund, G.G., Rahn, K.A., Nakamura, M.T., Yudell, B.E. A Reduced Carbohydrate, Increased Protein Diet Stabilizes Glycemic Control and Minimizes Adipose Tissue Glucose Disposal in Rats. *Journal of Nutrition*, July 1, 2006; 136(7); 1855-1861.

8.   Baum, J.I., Seyler, J.E., O'Conner, J.C., Freund, G.G., Layman, D.K. (2003). The effect of leucine on glucose homeostasis and the insulin signaling pathway. *FASEB J.* 17:A811.

9.   Bethesda, MD: National Institutes of Health, U.S. Department of Health and Human Services. What are adult stem cells? *Stem Cell Information* [World Wide Web site]. 2015 [cited Sunday, March 27, 2016] Available at http://stemcells.nih.gov/info/basics/pages/basics4.aspx

10. Brandhorst, S., Choi, I., Wei, M., Cheng, C., Sedrakyan, S., Navarrete, G., . . . Longo, V. (2015). A Periodic Diet that Mimics Fasting Promotes Multi-System Regeneration, Enhanced Cognitive Performance, and Healthspan. *Cell Metabolism, 22*(1), 86-99. doi:10.1016/j.cmet.2015.05.012

11. Bruce-Keller, A. J., Umberger, G., Mcfall, R., & Mattson, M. P. (1999). Food restriction reduces brain damage and improves behavioral outcome following excitotoxic and metabolic insults. *Annals of Neurology Ann Neurol., 45*(1), 8-15. doi:10.1002/1531-8249(199901)45:13.0.co;2-v

12. Calabrese, F., Rossetti, A. C., Racagni, G., Gass, P., Riva, M. A., & Molteni, R. (2014). Brain-derived neurotrophic factor: A bridge between inflammation and neuroplasticity. Frontiers in Cellular Neuroscience Front. Cell. Neurosci., 8. doi:10.3389/fncel.2014.00430

13. Carlson, O., Martin, B., Stote, K. S., Golden, E., Maudsley, S., Najjar, S. S., . . . Mattson, M. P. (2007). Impact of reduced meal frequency without caloric restriction on glucose regulation in healthy, normal-weight middle-aged men and women. *Metabolism, 56*(12), 1729-1734. doi:10.1016/j.metabol.2007.07.018

14. Chaix, A., Zarrinpar, A., Miu, P., & Panda, S. (2014). Time-Restricted Feeding Is a Preventative and Therapeutic Intervention against Diverse Nutritional Challenges. *Cell Metabolism, 20*(6), 991-1005. doi:10.1016/j.cmet.2014.11.001

15. Chaston, T. B., Dixon, J. B., & O'brien, P. E. (2006). Changes in fat-free mass during significant weight loss: A systematic review. *Int J Obes Relat Metab Disord International Journal of Obesity.* doi:10.1038/sj.ijo.0803483

16. Cheng, C., Adams, G., Perin, L., Wei, M., Zhou, X., Lam, B., . . . Longo, V. (2014). Prolonged Fasting Reduces IGF-1/PKA to Promote Hematopoietic-Stem-Cell-Based Regeneration and Reverse Immunosuppression. *Cell Stem Cell, 14*(6), 810-823. doi:10.1016/j.stem.2014.04.014

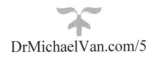

17. Daghestani, M. H. (2009). A preprandial and postprandial plasma levels of ghrelin hormone in lean, overweight and obese Saudi females. *Journal of King Saud University - Science, 21*(2), 119-124. doi:10.1016/j.jksus.2009.05.001

18. Deldicque, L., Bock, K. D., Maris, M., Ramaekers, M., Nielens, H., Francaux, M., & Hespel, P. (2009). Increased p70s6k phosphorylation during intake of a protein–carbohydrate drink following resistance exercise in the fasted state. European Journal of Applied Physiology Eur J Appl Physiol, 108(4), 791-800. doi:10.1007/s00421-009-1289-x

19. Descamps, O., Riondel, J., Ducros, V., & Roussel, A. (2005). Mitochondrial production of reactive oxygen species and incidence of age-associated lymphoma in OF1 mice: Effect of alternate-day fasting. *Mechanisms of Ageing and Development, 126*(11), 1185-1191. doi:10.1016/j.mad.2005.06.007

20. Dhurandhar, E. J., Dawson, J., Alcorn, A., Larsen, L. H., Thomas, E. A., Cardel, M., . . . Allison, D. B. (2014). The effectiveness of breakfast recommendations on weight loss: A randomized controlled trial. *American Journal of Clinical Nutrition, 100*(2), 507-513. doi:10.3945/ajcn.114.089573

21. Diano, S., Farr, S. A., Benoit, S. C., Mcnay, E. C., Silva, I. D., Horvath, B., . . . Horvath, T. L. (2006). Ghrelin controls hippocampal spine synapse density and memory performance. *Nature Neuroscience Nat Neurosci, 9*(3), 381-388. doi:10.1038/nn1656

22. Duan, W., & Mattson, M. P. (1999). Dietary restriction and 2-deoxyglucose administration improve behavioral outcome and reduce degeneration of dopaminergic neurons in models of Parkinson's disease. *J. Neurosci. Res. Journal of Neuroscience Research, 57*(2), 195-206. doi:10.1002/(sici)1097-4547(19990715)57:23.3.co;2-g

23. El-Khoury, A.E., Kukagawa, N.K., Sanchez, M., Tsay. R.H, Gleason, R.E., Chapman, T.E., Young. V.R. (1994). The 24-h pattern and rate of leucine oxidation, with particular reference to tracer estimates of leucine requirements in healthy adults. *Am. J. Clin. Nutr.* 59:1012-1020.

24. Evans, W. J., & Lexell, J. (1995). Human Aging, Muscle Mass, and Fiber Type Composition. *The Journals of Gerontology Series A: Biological Sciences and Medical Sciences, 50A*(Special), 11-16. doi:10.1093/gerona/50a.special_issue.11

25. Faris, A., Kacimi, S., Al-Kurd, R. A., Fararjeh, M. A., Bustanji, Y. K., Mohammad, M. K., & Salem, M. L. (2012). Intermittent fasting during Ramadan attenuates proinflammatory cytokines and immune cells in healthy subjects. Nutrition Research, 32(12), 947-955. doi:10.1016/j.nutres.2012.06.021

26. Fasting triggers stem cell regeneration of damaged, old immune system. (n.d.). Retrieved July 25, 2016, from http://news.usc.edu/63669/fasting-triggers-stem-cell-regeneration-of-damaged-old-immune-system/

27. Fernandes, G., Yunis, E. J., & Good, R. A. (1976). Influence of diet on survival of mice. *Proceedings of the National Academy of Sciences, 73*(4), 1279-1283. doi:10.1073/pnas.73.4.1279

28. Fiebig, R., Gore, M. T., Chandwaney, R., Leeuwenburgh, C., & Ji, L. L. (1996). Alteration of myocardial antioxidant enzyme activity and glutathione content with aging and exercise training. *Age, 19*(3), 83-89. doi:10.1007/bf02434087

29. Garlick, P.J. The Role of Leucine in the Regulation of Protein Metabolism. *Journal of Nutrition*, June 1, 2005; 135(6): 1553S-1556S.

30. Goodrick, C. L., Ingram, D. K., Reynolds, M. A., Freeman, J. R., & Cider, N. L. (2009). Effects of Intermittent Feeding Upon Growth and Life Span in Rats. *Gerontology, 28*(4), 233-241. doi:10.1159/000212538

31. Gøtzsche, P. C., & Jørgensen, K. J. (2013). Screening for breast cancer with mammography. *Cochrane Database of Systematic Reviews Reviews.* doi:10.1002/14651858.cd001877.pub5

32. Guyenet, S. J., & Schwartz, M. W. (2012). Regulation of Food Intake, Energy Balance, and Body Fat Mass: Implications for the Pathogenesis and Treatment of Obesity. The Journal of Clinical Endocrinology & Metabolism, 97(3), 745-755. doi:10.1210/jc.2011-2525

33. Halagappa, V. K., Guo, Z., Pearson, M., Matsuoka, Y., Cutler, R. G., Laferla, F. M., & Mattson, M. P. (2007). Intermittent fasting and caloric restriction ameliorate age-related behavioral deficits in the triple-transgenic mouse model of Alzheimer's disease. *Neurobiology of Disease, 26*(1), 212-220. doi:10.1016/j.nbd.2006.12.019

34. Halberg, N. (2005). Effect of intermittent fasting and refeeding on insulin action in healthy men. Journal of Applied Physiology, 99(6), 2128-2136. doi:10.1152/japplphysiol.00683.2005

35. Hall DM, Oberley TD, Moseley PM, Buettner GR, Oberley LW, Weindruch R, Kregel KC. (2000). Caloric restriction improves thermotolerance and reduces hyperthermia-induced cellular damage in old rats. *FASEB J, 14*, 78–86.

36. Heilbronn LK, Smith SR, Martin CK, Anton SD, Ravussin E. Alternate-day fasting in nonobese subjects: effects on body weight, body composition, and energy metabolism. *Am J Clin Nutr*. 2005; 81: 69–73.

37. Hirsch, J., Hudgin, L.C., Leibel, R.L., Rosenbaum, M. (1998). Diet composition and energy balance in humans. *Am. J. Clin. Nutr.* 67: 551S-555S.

38. Insulin Basics. (n.d.). Retrieved July 25, 2016, from http://www.diabetes.org/living-with-diabetes/treatment-and-care/medication/insulin/insulin-basics.html

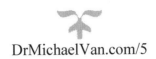

39. Johnson, J. B., Summer, W., Cutler, R. G., Martin, B., Hyun, D., Dixit, V. D., . . . Mattson, M. P. (2007). Alternate day calorie restriction improves clinical findings and reduces markers of oxidative stress and inflammation in overweight adults with moderate asthma. *Free Radical Biology and Medicine, 42*(5), 665-674. doi:10.1016/j.freeradbiomed.2006.12.005

40. Johnstone, A. (2014). Fasting for weight loss: An effective strategy or latest dieting trend? *Int J Obes Relat Metab Disord International Journal of Obesity, 39*(5), 727-733. doi:10.1038/ijo.2014.214

41. Kimball, S. R., & Jefferson, L. S. (2001). Regulation of protein synthesis by branched-chain amino acids. *Current Opinion in Clinical Nutrition and Metabolic Care, 4*(1), 39-43. doi:10.1097/00075197-200101000-00008

42. Klein, P., Tyrlikova, I., & Mathews, G. C. (2014). Dietary treatment in adults with refractory epilepsy: A review. *Neurology, 83*(21), 1978-1985. doi:10.1212/wnl.0000000000001004

43. Klempel, M. C., Kroeger, C. M., & Varady, K. A. (2013). Alternate day fasting (ADF) with a high-fat diet produces similar weight loss and cardio-protection as ADF with a low-fat diet. *Metabolism, 62*(1), 137-143. doi:10.1016/j.metabol.2012.07.002

44. Klok, M. D., Jakobsdottir, S., & Drent, M. L. (2007). The role of leptin and ghrelin in the regulation of food intake and body weight in humans: A review. *Obesity Reviews, 8*(1), 21-34. doi:10.1111/j.1467-789x.2006.00270.x

45. Kojima, M., Hosoda, H., & Kangawa, K. (2004). Ghrelin, a novel growth-hormone-releasing and appetite-stimulating peptide from stomach. *Best Practice & Research Clinical Endocrinology & Metabolism, 18*(4), 517-530. doi:10.1016/j.beem.2004.07.001

46. Koopman, R., & Loon, L. J. (2009). Aging, exercise, and muscle protein metabolism. *Journal of Applied Physiology, 106*(6), 2040-2048. doi:10.1152/japplphysiol.91551.2008

47. Krebs, M., Krssak, M., Bernroider, E., Anderwald, C., Brehm, A., Meyerspeer, M., . . . Roden, M. (2002). Mechanism of Amino Acid-Induced Skeletal Muscle Insulin Resistance in Humans. *Diabetes, 51*(3), 599-605. doi:10.2337/diabetes.51.3.599

48. Layman, D. K. (2002). Role of Leucine in Protein Metabolism During Exercise and Recovery. *Canadian Journal of Applied Physiology Can. J. Appl. Physiol., 27*(6), 646-662. doi:10.1139/h02-038

49. Layman, D. K., Evans, E. M., Erickson, D., Seyler, J., Weber, J., Bagshaw, D., . . . Kris-Etherton, P. (2009). A Moderate-Protein Diet Produces Sustained Weight Loss and Long-Term Changes in Body Composition and Blood Lipids in Obese Adults. *Journal of Nutrition, 139*(3), 514-521. doi:10.3945/jn.108.099440

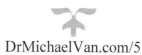

50.   Layman, D.K. (2003). The role of leucine in weight loss diets and glucose homeostasis. *Journal of Nutrition.* 133:261S-267S.

51.   Layman, D.K., Baum, J.I. (2004). Dietary Protein Impact on Glycemic Control during Weight Loss. The American Society for Nutritional Sciences. *Journal of Nutrition.* 134:968S-973S, April 2004.

52.   Layman, D.K., Baum, J.I. (2004). The Emerging Role of Dairy Proteins and Bioactive Peptides in Nutrition and Health. The American Society for Nutritional Sciences. *Journal of Nutrition.* 134:968S-973S, April 2004.

53.   Layman, D.K., Walker, D.A. Potential Importance of Leucine in Treatment of Obesity and the Metabolic Syndrome. *Journal of Nutrition*, January 1, 2006; 136(1): 319S-323S.

54.   Layman. D.K., Boileau, R.A., Erickson. D.J., Painter, J.E., Shiue, H., Sather, C., Christou, D.D. (2003). A reduced ratio of dietary carbohydrate to protein improves body composition and blood lipid profiles during weight loss in men. *Journal of Nutrition.* 133:411-417.

55.   Layman. D.K., Shiue, H., Sather, C., Erickson, D.J., Baum, J. (2003). Increased dietary protein modifies glucose and insulin homeostasis in adult women during weight loss. *Journal of Nutrition.* 133:405-410.

56.   Lee, C., Raffaghello, L., Brandhorst, S., Safdie, F. M., Bianchi, G., Martin-Montalvo, A., . . . Longo, V. D. (2012). Fasting Cycles Retard Growth of Tumors and Sensitize a Range of Cancer Cell Types to Chemotherapy. *Science Translational Medicine, 4*(124). doi:10.1126/scitranslmed.3003293

57.   Lee, G. D., Wilson, M. A., Zhu, M., Wolkow, C. A., Cabo, R. D., Ingram, D. K., & Zou, S. (2006). Dietary deprivation extends lifespan in Caenorhabditis elegans. *Aging Cell, 5*(6), 515-524. doi:10.1111/j.1474-9726.2006.00241.x

58.   Lemon, P. W. (2000). Beyond the Zone: Protein Needs of Active Individuals. *Journal of the American College of Nutrition, 19*(Sup5). doi:10.1080/07315724.2000.10718974

59.   Lexell, J., & Downham, D. (1992). What is the effect of ageing on type 2 muscle fibres? *Journal of the Neurological Sciences, 107*(2), 250-251. doi:10.1016/0022-510x(92)90297-x

60.   Lu, X. (2007). The leptin hypothesis of depression: A potential link between mood disorders and obesity? Current Opinion in Pharmacology, 7(6), 648-652. doi:10.1016/j.coph.2007.10.010

61.   Lutter, M., Sakata, I., Osborne-Lawrence, S., Rovinsky, S. A., Anderson, J. G., Jung, S., . . . Zigman, J. M. (2008). The orexigenic hormone ghrelin defends against depressive symptoms of chronic stress. *Nature Neuroscience Nat Neurosci, 11*(7), 752-753. doi:10.1038/nn.2139

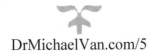

DrMichaelVan.com/5

62.   Marx, J. O., Kraemer, W. J., Nindl, B. C., & Larsson, L. (2002). Effects of Aging on Human Skeletal Muscle Myosin Heavy-Chain mRNA Content and Protein Isoform Expression. *The Journals of Gerontology Series A: Biological Sciences and Medical Sciences, 57*(6). doi:10.1093/gerona/57.6.b232

63.   Mattson, M. P. (2005). The need for controlled studies of the effects of meal frequency on health. *The Lancet, 365*(9475), 1978-1980. doi:10.1016/s0140-6736(05)66667-6

64.   Mattson, M. P. (2008). Dietary factors, hormesis and health. *Ageing Research Reviews, 7*(1), 43-48. doi:10.1016/j.arr.2007.08.004

65.   Mattson, M. P., Allison, D. B., Fontana, L., Harvie, M., Longo, V. D., Malaisse, W. J., . . . Panda, S. (2014). Meal frequency and timing in health and disease. *Proceedings of the National Academy of Sciences Proc Natl Acad Sci USA, 111*(47), 16647-16653. doi:10.1073/pnas.1413965111

66.   Mattson, M., & Wan, R. (2005). Beneficial effects of intermittent fasting and caloric restriction on the cardiovascular and cerebrovascular systems. The Journal of Nutritional Biochemistry, 16(3), 129-137. doi:10.1016/j.jnutbio.2004.12.007

67.   Michalsen, A., Riegert, M., Lüdtke, R., Bäcker, M., Langhorst, J., Schwickert, M., & Dobos, G. J. (2005). Mediterranean diet or extended fasting's influence on changing the intestinal microflora, immunoglobulin A secretion and clinical outcome in patients with rheumatoid arthritis and fibromyalgia: An observational study. *BMC Complementary and Alternative Medicine BMC Complement Altern Med, 5*(1). doi:10.1186/1472-6882-5-22

68.   Miller, A. B., Wall, C., Baines, C. J., Sun, P., To, T., & Narod, S. A. (2014). Twenty five year follow-up for breast cancer incidence and mortality of the Canadian National Breast Screening Study: Randomised screening trial. *Bmj, 348*(Feb11 9). doi:10.1136/bmj.g366

69.   Norton, L.E., Layman, D.K. Leucine Regulates Translation Initiation of Protein Synthesis in Skeletal Muscle after Exercise. *Journal of Nutrition*, February 1, 2006; 136(2); 533S-537S.

70.   Paddon-Jones, D. (2003). Amino acid ingestion improves muscle protein synthesis in the young and elderly. *AJP: Endocrinology and Metabolism, 286*(3). doi:10.1152/ajpendo.00368.2003

71.   Poff, A., Ari, C., Arnold, P., Seyfried, T., & D'agostino, D. (2014). Ketone supplementation decreases tumor cell viability and prolongs survival of mice with metastatic cancer. *International Journal of Cancer Int. J. Cancer, 135*(7), 1711-1720. doi:10.1002/ijc.28809

72. Putman, C., Hollidge-Horvath, M., Lands, L., Lukezic, T., Jones, N., & Heigenhauser, G. (1994). Pyruvate Dehydrogenase Activity and Acetyl-Group Accumulation in Human Vastus Lateralis during Maximal Intermittent Isokinetic Cycling. *Clin. Sci. Clinical Science, 87*(S1), 58-59. doi:10.1042/cs087s058

73. Reeds, P., Burrin, D., Davis, T., & Stoll, B. (1998). Amino acid metabolism and the energetics of growth. *Archiv Für Tierernaehrung, 51*(2-3), 187-197. doi:10.1080/17450399809381918

74. Rennie, M.J, Tipton, K. D. (2000). Protein and amino acid metabolism during and after exercise and the effects of nutrition. *Annu. Rev. Nutr.* 20:457-483.

75. Rocha, N. S., Barbisan, L. F., Oliveira, M. L., & Camargo, J. L. (2002). Effects of fasting and intermittent fasting on rat hepatocarcinogenesis induced by diethylnitrosamine. *Teratog. Carcinog. Mutagen. Teratogenesis, Carcinogenesis, and Mutagenesis, 22*(2), 129-138. doi:10.1002/tcm.10005

76. Rosenfeldt, M. T., & Ryan, K. M. (2011). The multiple roles of autophagy in cancer. *Carcinogenesis, 32*(7), 955-963. doi:10.1093/carcin/bgr031

77. Ruderman, N. B. (1975). Muscle Amino Acid Metabolism and Gluconeogenesis. *Annual Review of Medicine Annu. Rev. Med., 26*(1), 245-258. doi:10.1146/annurev.me.26.020175.001333

78. Sanz, A., Pamplona, R., & Barja, G. (2006). Is the Mitochondrial Free Radical Theory of Aging Intact? *Antioxidants & Redox Signaling, 8*(3-4), 582-599. doi:10.1089/ars.2006.8.582

79. Shapiro, A., Mu, W., Roncal, C., Cheng, K., Johnson, R. J., & Scarpace, P. J. (2008). Fructose-induced leptin resistance exacerbates weight gain in response to subsequent high-fat feeding. AJP: Regulatory, Integrative and Comparative Physiology, 295(5). doi:10.1152/ajpregu.00195.2008

80. Shiiya, T., Nakazato, M., Mizuta, M., Date, Y., Mondal, M. S., Tanaka, M., . . . Matsukura, S. (2002). Plasma Ghrelin Levels in Lean and Obese Humans and the Effect of Glucose on Ghrelin Secretion. *The Journal of Clinical Endocrinology & Metabolism, 87*(1), 240-244. doi:10.1210/jcem.87.1.8129

81. Short, K. R. (2003). Age and aerobic exercise training effects on whole body and muscle protein metabolism. *AJP: Endocrinology and Metabolism, 286*(1). doi:10.1152/ajpendo.00366.2003

82. Siegel, I., Liu, T. L., Nepomuceno, N., & Gleicher, N. (1988). Effects of Short-Term Dietary Restriction on Survival of Mammary Ascites Tumor-Bearing Rats. *Cancer Investigation, 6*(6), 677-680. doi:10.3109/07357908809078034

83. Simopoulos, A. P. (2005). What Is So Special about the Diet of Greece? The Scientific Evidence. *Nutrition and Fitness: Mental Health, Aging, and the Implementation of a Healthy Diet and Physical Activity Lifestyle World Review of Nutrition and Dietetics,* 80-92. doi:10.1159/000088275

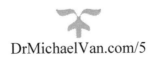

84. Sinha, M. K., Opentanova, I., Ohannesian, J. P., Kolaczynski, J. W., Heiman, M. L., Hale, J., . . . Caro, J. F. (1996). Evidence of free and bound leptin in human circulation. Studies in lean and obese subjects and during short-term fasting. Journal of Clinical Investigation J. Clin. Invest., 98(6), 1277-1282. doi:10.1172/jci118913

85. Skov, A. R., Toubro, S., Rønn, B., Holm, L., & Astrup, A. (1999). Randomized trial on protein vs carbohydrate in ad libitum fat reduced diet for the treatment of obesity. *Int J Obes Relat Metab Disord International Journal of Obesity, 23*(5), 528-536. doi:10.1038/sj.ijo.0800867

86. Staron, R. S., Malicky, E. S., Leonardi, M. J., Falkel, J. E., Hagerman, F. C., & Dudley, G. A. (1990). Muscle hypertrophy and fast fiber type conversions in heavy resistance-trained women. *European Journal of Applied Physiology and Occupational Physiology Europ. J. Appl. Physiol., 60*(1), 71-79. doi:10.1007/bf00572189

87. Stipp, D. (2015). Is Fasting Good for You? *Sci Am Scientific American, 24*(1s), 56-57. doi:10.1038/scientificamericansecrets0315-56

88. Stote KS et al. (2007). A controlled trial of reduced meal frequency without caloric restriction in healthy, normal-weight, middle-aged adults. *Am J Clin Nutr, 85*(4), 981-88.

89. Svanberg, E., Jefferson, L.S., Lundhold, K., Kimball, S.R. (1997). Postprandial stimulation of muscle protein synthesis is independent of changes in insulin. *Endocrinology and Metabolism*, Vol. 272, Issue 5 E841-E847.

90. Thaler, J. P., Yi, C., Schur, E. A., Guyenet, S. J., Hwang, B. H., Dietrich, M. O., . . . Schwartz, M. W. (2012). Obesity is associated with hypothalamic injury in rodents and humans. Journal of Clinical Investigation J. Clin. Invest., 122(1), 153-162. doi:10.1172/jci59660

91. The American Journal of Clinical Nutrition. (n.d.). Retrieved July 25, 2016, from http://ajcn.nutrition.org/content/87/5/1576S.full

92. Torrazza, R. M., Suryawan, A., Gazzaneo, M. C., Orellana, R. A., Frank, J. W., Nguyen, H. V., . . . Davis, T. A. (2010). Leucine Supplementation of a Low-Protein Meal Increases Skeletal Muscle and Visceral Tissue Protein Synthesis in Neonatal Pigs by Stimulating mTOR-Dependent Translation Initiation. *Journal of Nutrition, 140*(12), 2145-2152. doi:10.3945/jn.110.128421

93. Tschop, M., Weyer, C., Tataranni, P. A., Devanarayan, V., Ravussin, E., & Heiman, M. L. (2001). Circulating Ghrelin Levels Are Decreased in Human Obesity. *Diabetes, 50*(4), 707-709. doi:10.2337/diabetes.50.4.707

94. Varady KA, Allister CA, Hellerstein MK. Effect of alternate day fasting on lipid metabolism in obese humans. Unpublished data.

95. Varady KA, Bhutani S, Klempel MC, Kroeger C. Effect of alternate day fasting combined with exercise on body composition parameters in obese adults. Unpublished data.

96.   Varady, K. A. (2011). Intermittent versus daily calorie restriction: Which diet regimen is more effective for weight loss? *Obesity Reviews, 12*(7). doi:10.1111/j.1467-789x.2011.00873.x

97.   Varady, K. A., Bhutani, S., Church, E. C., & Klempel, M. C. (2009). Short-term modified alternate-day fasting: A novel dietary strategy for weight loss and cardioprotection in obese adults. American Journal of Clinical Nutrition, 90(5), 1138-1143. doi:10.3945/ajcn.2009.28380

98.   Vasselli, J. R., Weindruch, R., Heymsfield, S. B., Pi-Sunyer, F. X., Boozer, C. N., Yi, N., . . . Allison, D. B. (2005). Intentional Weight Loss Reduces Mortality Rate in a Rodent Model of Dietary Obesity. *Obesity Research, 13*(4), 693-702. doi:10.1038/oby.2005.78

99.   Wagenmakers, A. J. (1998). 11 Muscle Amino Acid Metabolism at Rest and During Exercise. *Exercise and Sport Sciences Reviews, 26.* doi:10.1249/00003677-199800260-00013

100. Welch, H. G., & Passow, H. J. (2014). Quantifying the Benefits and Harms of Screening Mammography. *JAMA Internal Medicine JAMA Intern Med, 174*(3), 448. doi:10.1001/jamainternmed.2013.13635

101. Wu, G., & Morris, S. M. (1998). Arginine metabolism: Nitric oxide and beyond. *Biochem. J. Biochemical Journal, 336*(1), 1-17. doi:10.1042/bj3360001

102. Wu, J., Liu, J., Chen, E., Wang, J., Cao, L., Narayan, N., . . . Finkel, T. (2013). Increased Mammalian Lifespan and a Segmental and Tissue-Specific Slowing of Aging after Genetic Reduction of mTOR Expression. *Cell Reports, 4*(5), 913-920. doi:10.1016/j.celrep.2013.07.030